ENCYCLOPEDIA OF

ALLERGY AND ENVIRONMENTAL ILLNESS

A SELF-HELP APPROACH

ELLEN ROTHERA

David & Charles

British Library Cataloguing-in-Publication Data

Rothera, Ellen
    Encyclopedia of allergy and environmental illness
    A self-help approach.
    I. Title
    616.97

    ISBN 0-7153-9876-8 (hbk)
    ISBN 0-7153-9954-3 (pbk)

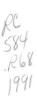
© Ellen Rothera 1991

Typeset by XL Publishing Services, Nairn, Scotland
and printed in Hong Kong
by Wing King Tong Co Ltd
for David & Charles plc
Brunel House   Newton Abbot   Devon

CONTENTS

ACKNOWLEDGEMENTS

I dedicate this book to my husband David, who must at times have wished he had chosen a more conventional wife, but has never actually said so and is what Bertie Wooster would have described as a 'good egg'.

. . . . . .

I wish to express my grateful thanks to the following:

John Button, my agent, who was helpful and reassuring and convinced me I could write this book; my husband David, who gave me his unfailing support and encouragement; Dr James Anderson, who kindly checked over the medical facts and terminology and advised accordingly; Ann Faulkner, who provided me with valuable information regarding anaesthetics; Brenda O'Reilly of the Allergy-Induced Autism and Self Help Group, who allowed me to publish her own material on the subject; Dr Eric Millstone, for permitting me to quote him on the subject of additives; Amelia Nathan Hill of Action Against Allergy and Eunice Rose of the National Society of Research into Allergy, who helped me with research; my daughter Sally, who, in her professional role of research assistant, interpreted the research and put it into lay terms; Maureen Smith, who typed the manuscript so professionally; my daughter Deborah, who helped sort out a last-minute panic, thereby enabling me to meet my deadline; Faith Glasgow and Alison Elks who, on behalf of David & Charles kept the wheels running smoothly.

I should also like to thank the chemist who allowed me to publish his personal experiences; the associations and individuals whose names I have been permitted to include, and all those people who have provided me with most valuable snippets of information along the way.

FOREWORD

In this book I have tried to cover all the questions I have been asked over a number of years; these questions range from advice on pregnancy, allergic babies, weaning, hyperactivity and other allergies in children to all the many and varied manifestations of allergic illness in adults – including myalgic encephalomyelitis (ME), which is a severe form of multiple allergies.

It has been well said that being an allergic person is a life problem as much as a health problem as we each inherit our own degree of susceptibility, and it is from this angle that I have approached the subject. There are already many excellent books on allergies (and some not so good), but perhaps not too many have been written by people who have suffered to a great extent and have managed totally to stabilise their condition. That I have had the good fortune to be able to do so seemed sufficient reason for passing on information which has taken me years to accumulate.

Whether you are a sufferer, or a parent of a sufferer, or whether you require information for a project or other purpose, all I know is collated in this book. It includes a list of allergy associations any of which you may join if you so desire. They will provide you with additional information, including names of doctors working in this field. I do not know how much longer I shall be able to continue running my association therefore I hope that this encyclopedia will help, in some small part, to fulfil the need which clearly exists to provide information on allergies.

My heart goes out to all of you, so often maligned and misunderstood, in your search for practical help and the means to put it into action. I hope this book will give you hope and encouragement.

Believe me, with the right knowledge and sufficient willpower, there is relief to be found for everyone.

Ellen Rothera

INTRODUCTION

If you are suffering from some type of infection, the chances are that sooner or later a member of the medical profession will make a diagnosis and offer you whatever treatment is available.

If you need surgery, you can hope to be operated on in the not-too-distant future.

If you have a baby, all your needs will be catered for in hospital, if you so desire, and those of your baby also.

If you are involved in an accident, then you can be taken to your nearest accident department (provided at most major hospitals).

All this at no extra cost! Unless we choose otherwise. What a wonderful service is provided for us in this country! (Those who disagree should try a spell of living abroad.)

It is only in the area of chronic illness that the medical profession so often falls down and people are forced to look elsewhere for help. So much chronic illness – either constant or of a recurring nature – is environmentally induced. Find the cause and you can remove the symptoms! This should be possible for most people to achieve, providing they are prepared to work at it.

So many people are distressed because they have been told that they are neurotic and made to feel responsible for their own symptoms. In my opinion, most people are far too busy trying to run their daily lives to have time to be neurotic. I believe that this inference is a common reaction in doctors who are at a loss as to how to help their patients, and this is a convenient way of passing on the responsibility. I doubt whether they realise just how much distress this attitude can cause. Still one of the major hurdles allergic people face is the lack of understanding of those not similarly afflicted.

A person who is in a generally low state, for whatever reason, is more susceptible than he otherwise would be. Very stressful situations, such as bereavements, can make someone temporarily more susceptible. Coming to terms with the stress will be as important in the recovery as discovering the allergens.

Some major stresses which may trigger the development of allergies are imbalance of hormones, infection, prolonged or severe environmental stress, shock, nutritional inadequacy of minerals and vitamins, repeated doses of antibiotics or other drugs and exposure to chemicals.

We live in an ever-increasingly polluted and stressful world and many people's bodies have gone into 'overload'. In other words, our bodies have reached chemical saturation point. This damages the immune system which alters the body chemistry and causes a variety of (possibly random) symptoms to appear. None of this is so surprising when you learn, for example, that (i) the average child of five today is said already to have consumed seven pounds of chemical additives, only some of which will have been eliminated, and (ii) nowadays when people die their bodies stay unnaturally preserved due to all the preservatives they have consumed. Taking regular vitamin and mineral supplements helps to prevent the build-up of a toxic overload.

For those who know or suspect that they suffer from chemical sensitivities, the following questionnaire is worth consideration. All those questions to which you answer 'yes' must be regarded as indicating possible causes. It is unlikely that even the most sensitive people will react to all of them but each item listed is suspect until proven otherwise.

Do you smoke?
Do any members of your family smoke?
Is your house damp?
Has your house been treated for damp?
Do you – or other members of your family – use scented toiletries such as soaps, talcs, deodorants etc?
Do you use perfume/after-shave?
Do you use perfumed hair sprays or perfumed cleaning materials?
Do you have a gas/oil-fired boiler?
Do you come into contact with chemicals at home/work/school?
Do your colleagues/friends smoke or use perfume?
Has your home been chemically treated (ie cavity wall insulation, wood preservatives, carpets professionally cleaned, interior recently painted or treated for woodworm etc)?
Do you have gas fires or a gas cooker?
Do you use chemicals in your garden?
Do you live in a built-up area where you come into contact with car or factory fumes?
Do you live near fields or a nursery garden where aerial spraying may be done?

Apart from chemicals and the well-known house dust and house-dust mite, other sources of allergy in the home are house plants and cut flowers which can cause breathing, eye, nasal and skin problems.

If your symptoms do not appear to be related to the environment you will doubtless be turning to your diet for inspiration. The first chapter covers the subject in detail.

This encyclopedia provides a guide only to some of the most likely causes, where these are known, of allergy-induced symptoms. Each and every one can also be caused by other illnesses, some of them serious. Therefore, the advice and recommendations should be used only if your doctor has declared that he can find no other reason for your symptoms and that it is neither his nor your wish for you to be referred elsewhere. I should like to point out that where I have used terms such as 'foods which have been implicated' I am referring to those which I have uncovered in my research. Allergy is such an individual matter that it is quite within the realms of possibility for *anyone* to be allergic to *anything*.

I cannot guarantee to have covered every possible allergy symptom in the following pages so, if you are suffering from something which is *not* listed, please do not discount the possibility that it might *still* be of allergic origin.

Good reading and good luck!

CHAPTER 1

COMMON FOOD ALLERGENS

The difference between a food allergy and a food intolerance is that in an allergy the patient has a reaction within anything from a few minutes to twenty-four hours. The reaction may be severe even when only a small amount of food or drink has been consumed. Intolerances are caused by the build-up of the effects of a food over a period of days. It may even be necessary for such a food to have been eaten in fairly large quantities before symptoms become obvious. Intolerances are usually caused by foods we eat very regularly – such as wheat, milk, eggs and yeast. These are common food allergens, too, but the range of other possibilities is much wider in food allergy. In food intolerance the symptoms are not usually constant, and a tolerance can more easily be regained.

MILK

Probably the most common of all food allergens is cow's milk. It has almost three times the protein content of human milk and it is the protein in foods which usually causes the allergic reaction. A fair proportion of babies are sensitive to it, causing problems which show up regularly in the form of eczema and colic.

Another reason why people can be sensitive to cow's milk is that cows are given a maintenance dose of antibiotic, and some of them are treated with hormones; thus, we may be reacting to these substances. Unigate have a pilot scheme in the Torbay area of Devon where 'green' pints are being delivered. In order to produce this organic milk, grazing meadows are left fallow for two years and no chemical or artificial treatments are used. The fields are fertilised naturally by the cows which have been grazing on organic grass. It all seems so obvious!

Those people who cannot tolerate cow's milk may find that they can take goat's or ewe's milk. The latter can be bought frozen from many health food shops. Some people will have problems even with these or, from preference, may choose soya milk. This comes in either a sweetened or unsweetened form and is considered by many to be a very satisfactory substitute. It can be used in any way in which cow's milk would be used and, being of a slightly thicker consistency, can be diluted when used for custards and other sauces. It does not naturally contain calcium so it is a good idea to consider taking a calcium supplement. The exception to this is in soya-based baby formulas in which calcium has been specially added.

In the following pages, where milk is listed as a common cause of any particular symptom, I have not felt it necessary to add each time the words 'and milk products'. However, if you are eliminating cow's milk from your diet, it is also essential to cut out anything made from it as well, such as cheese, butter, yoghurt, ice cream etc.

If you are sensitive to cow's milk, you may find the following information useful – depending on your degree of sensitivity. Milk heated to a very high temperature – such as evaporated milk – loses some of its allergenic properties, so some people will be able to tolerate it in this form. Others may find it more easily tolerated as yoghurt. People who react to the whey of the milk (which contains the protein, casein) may find that they can take a thick cream or a hard cheese (but not a soft cheese). Others who react to the cream of the milk, or who have a problem in the digestion of fats, will find the situation reversed. Yet again, there will be those who cannot tolerate milk except in the form of a *cooked* cheese

Whereas milk-allergic people may never be able to tolerate cheese, cheese-allergic people are not necessarily allergic to milk! This is because the process required to turn milk into cheese has altered its chemical properties. Hard cheeses, for example, contain tyramine, which causes some people to have headaches or migraine, so it may be this which is causing their symptoms and not the milk protein. For this reason cheese has been entered as a separate item under the list of possible causes in the Encyclopedia. Goat's or ewe's cheese should be satisfactory for those people who can tolerate goat's or ewe's milk. So you see, there are many options you can experiment with once you have left cow's milk out of your diet for a while and given your body a chance to regain a tolerance.

GRAINS

Wheat is by far the most common allergen amongst the grains. One reason is that we eat so much of it, so often (some people consume it at every meal), that our bodies can become sensitised to it. In some cases people may be reacting to the mould-killing sprays used before harvesting. Others may be reacting to the benzoyl chloride which is used as a bleaching agent for white flour before milling. Then there are the many artificial additives which bakers may use prior to baking. Those people who have problems with additives may find that wholemeal bread baked in home bakeries suits them best. The ingredients in the purest of loaves will consist of wholemeal flour, yeast, salt, water and a minute amount of emulsifier (with the possibility of other ingredients also). People who are affected by the yeast or the emulsifier, but are not wheat-sensitive, may choose to bake their own bread. For the yeast-sensitive, soda bread is bread made without yeast. Surprisingly, although the majority are likely to tolerate better the untampered-with wholemeal flour, I have met people who find they are better on white flour. They are unaffected by the bleaching process but are bran-sensitive.

Confusion sometimes arises when people are not sure of the difference between being wheat-sensitive and gluten-sensitive. Gluten is the main protein in wheat and is present also in rye and barley and, to a lesser extent, in oats. When we think of gluten-intolerance, we tend to think of coeliac disease, although it is quite possible to have a gluten-intolerance and suffer from other symptoms. So a wheat-sensitive person must avoid wheat in all its forms but may be able to eat rye, barley and oats; a gluten-sensitive person must avoid wheat, barley, rye and oats but should be able to tolerate these grains when the gluten has been removed. These people need to look for those products marked '100% gluten-free' – others marked only 'gluten-free' are misleading and may in fact contain a small amount of gluten which would be enough to cause a reaction in some people. Grains other than wheat, rye, barley and oats do *not* contain gluten and so it may be safer to do your own baking with alternative flours (of which there are many) obtainable from health food shops.

Now to the corn/maize question. Corn and maize are exactly the same thing. Cornflour, sweet corn and cornflakes are all maize. You will see maize listed as the main ingredient on a packet of cornflakes. The Americans always use the term corn, and they may be unfamiliar with the word maize.

CAFFEINE

You can be adversely affected by coffee, tea or chocolate, and this can be an individual allergic reaction. You can be affected by the chemical processing which changes the coffee bean into coffee powder (which is why some people are not affected by ground coffee but are affected by instant coffee) or which changes the tea plant into dried tea leaves.

You can have a bad reaction to cola drinks for a variety of reasons. One well-known brand lists its ingredients as carbonated water, sugar, colour-caramel, flavourings, orthophosphoric acid and caffeine. However, what they all have in common is caffeine and this is far more likely to cause most people's problems. A caffeine sensitivity is not so much an allergy as a lower threshold of caffeine toxity. Why is this? The reason is that caffeine is a drug, and a strong one at that. It is found naturally in tea, coffee and chocolate, and is added to cola drinks; it is also put into some over-the-counter drugs, usually pain-killers (*Anadin*, for example).

Caffeine acts upon the central nervous system very rapidly, and it gives an immediate 'lift' – which is why people so often become addicted, especially to coffee but also to tea. Unfortunately, when this effect wears off some people may become tense, nervous, fatigued, strained and, if they persist with topping up their daily intake, will probably start to lose weight as well. Insomnia is another not unexpected side-effect of constantly consuming a stimulant. Doctors believe that heavy coffee drinkers increase the risk of heart attacks and other serious conditions. They advise anyone who drinks five cups or more a day to cut down on their caffeine intake. It is much more difficult to give up smoking if you are a coffee drinker, incidentally.

Decaffeinated coffee is not recommended because the chemicals required for the decaffeination process have been found to cause additional problems. The only exception to this of which I am aware is Café Hag, which is decaffeinated over water rather than chemicals.

It has been my experience that some people who choose to give up coffee and tea seem to be at a loss as to what they can drink as substitutes. There are lots of alternatives to be found in health food shops – I name but some: Barleycup, Dandelion coffee, 'Postum', Luaka tea, Rooibosch tea and a wide variety of herb teas. You do need to check on herb teas, though, as some contain caffeine and others tannin. Some people are unable to tolerate even these drinks. You can also buy pure fruit juices which are very pleasant when diluted with water. (Do *not* buy fruit *squashes* which contain preservatives such as sodium metabisulphite which cause nasty problems, especially in children.) Also, don't forget, there is nothing wrong with lots and lots of lovely WATER (filtered if necessary).

EGGS

Eggs are another common source of allergy and can produce severe reactions in infants when given for the first time. For this reason the most common vaccines, which used to be cultured in egg, are now cultured in beef broth. The yolk and the white are chemically different and, as such, should be considered separately, although some people will not be able to tolerate either. The egg white, or albumen, is the protein and is the more likely culprit. Babies should be tried on a small amount of egg yolk initially. As with milk, when eggs are heated to a high enough temperature some of the allergenic properties are destroyed; therefore, hard-boiled eggs or eggs baked in cakes may be better tolerated by otherwise egg-allergic people. Some people are so allergic to eggs that they can suffer skin allergies through coming into contact with the shells – or may even be affected by the fumes of eggs as they are being cooked or by kissing someone who has recently eaten an egg.

FISH

People may be allergic to fish and some people can tolerate fish only when it is absolutely fresh. Those people who are allergic to fish can have severe reactions and may even produce symptoms from the fumes of fish as it is being cooked, or by touching fish (raw or cooked) or by kissing someone who has recently eaten it. Watch out for kippers and smoked mackerel which may contain the colouring Brown FK, and smoked cod and haddock, which, unless smoked naturally, will simply be coloured with tartrazine (E102), easily recognised by their vivid yellow colour. Shellfish come into a different category and are a common cause of allergies.

CHOCOLATE

Chocolate is quite a common allergen for a variety of reasons. It contains caffeine and is therefore a stimulant. It contains tyramine and phenylethylamine, common sources of allergen particularly to migraine sufferers. It seems that migraine sufferers may be deficient in certain enzymes thus causing an inability to metabolise these amino acids. Some chocolate-allergic people react to allergens contained in the whole cocoa bean. These people may be able to tolerate white chocolate providing they are not sensitive to any of the ingredients. The ingredients are likely to be cocoa butter (the fat fraction of the cocoa bean only), milk solids, sugar, vegetable fat, vanilla flavouring and, possibly, an emulsifier. An alternative to chocolate bars is carob bars (milk or plain). The carob bean is quite different from the cocoa bean and is tolerated by most people. You can buy it in either milk or plain bars or in powder form for drinks, and it is sold in health food shops.

MISCELLANEOUS FOODS

Peanuts are not nuts at all but belong to the legume family of plants along with peas, beans and lentils. Because of this they are classified separately from nuts in this book.

Citrus fruits include oranges, lemons, limes, tangerines, satsumas and grapefruit etc. Most books on allergy list them together under the heading 'citrus fruits', so I have done the same. However, because someone reacts to one it does not necessarily mean he reacts to the others. Oranges are the more likely culprits as most of us consume more of these than any other citrus fruit.

Sugar cane and sugar beet are quite different. Sugar cane belongs to the grass family, and sugar beet (believe it or not) belongs to the spinach family. Sucrose is another name for both sugars. Fructose is fruit sugar; lactose is milk sugar. Glucose and dextrose are derived from maize, as is corn syrup.

All honeys are different, depending upon where the bees collect them. For example, someone who is allergic to oranges may not be able to take honey which comes from orange blossom and so on. Most people can tolerate honey collected from heather.

Some salts, even sea salts, may contain sodium hexacyanoferrate II which is used as a pouring agent. (It is also used in the manufacture of some wines.) Some people will react to this chemical. It is preferable to look for sea salt which contains no additives at all.

With regard to alcohol, some people will be allergic to alcohol per se and others simply drink too much. However, many people are, unwittingly, affected by (and possibly addicted to) the constituent parts of alcohol. Most alcoholic drinks contain several ingredients.

Wines and sherries are commonly made from grapes. Red wine contains an amino acid called tyramine (as do chocolate and cheese) which cannot be metabolised by some people. It is one of the common causes of headaches and migraine. White wine is tyramine-free and most German white wines are usually free from artificial additives. Many of the cheaper wines contain up to twenty or so permitted additives. The ground in which the grapes have been grown may have been treated with chemicals, or the grapes may have been sprayed with chemicals several times throughout their growth. A wide range of organic wines is now available, and non-alcoholic ones are becoming increasingly popular.

Beer is made from hops but it contains other ingredients including corn, wheat, barley, rye and yeast. It is worth knowing that the components of beer can vary.

Gin is made from juniper, whiskey from wheat, barley or rye, and rum from cane sugar.

To sum up: all alcoholic drinks contain yeast, most contain sugar, and many contain artificial additives.

CHAPTER 2

FOOD ADDITIVES

Sometimes people are under a misconception as to what constitutes junk food. Fish and chips or beans and eggs are not junk food. Providing that they are part of a varied diet which contains plenty of fruit and vegetables (and any frying is done in vegetable fat, rather than animal fat) they are good forms of protein and carbohydrate.

Junk food is food which has been tampered with and/or had unnatural substances (which have been produced in a chemistry laboratory) added to it to enhance its colour, flavour etc. Apart from preservatives in tinned meat, none of this is strictly necessary as some more enterprising manufacturers have already proved. Typical junk food is cola, one brand of which contains carbonated water, sugar, caramel colouring, flavourings, orthophosphoric acid and caffeine.

Food additives continue to be produced because those who make them have convinced food manufacturers that they are necessary. This is in order to keep the additive manufacturers in business (and a very lucrative one at that). It is irrespective of the fact that most of us do not want them. As Erik Millstone states in his book, *Additives. A Guide For Everyone*: 'We believe ... that the benefit of doubt has consistently been awarded to industry and not to consumers where it rightfully belongs'. Some food additives are bad for some people and others are bad for everyone. The latter may not be immediately apparent but, over the years, they may cause, or contribute to, the development of cancer and other forms of degenerative disease. Some additives can inhibit the absorption of certain nutrients. Let me give you an example of two you are better off without. I assure you there are many others. The colouring 154 Brown FK, used for colouring smoked and cured fish, is under consideration for an E prefix despite doubts about its safety. It has been in constant use throughout the past thirty years. 513 Sulphuric acid is also under consideration for an E prefix despite the fact that it is poisonous! It is used to regulate acidity in the brewing industry and to modify starch.

Erik Millstone explained in 1990: 'the fact that a chemical additive has an E number is supposed to indicate that the European Community can vouch for the safety of the chemical bearing that number but, in practice, consumers cannot yet be confident that this assumption is valid. The European Scientific Committee for Food has not had time to review all the compounds on its lists. Not all the chemicals have been properly tested and evidence that they may cause problems has not always been taken sufficiently seriously'.

Synthetic chemicals in foods are usually derived from petroleum, coal tar or cellulose. Three or four pounds of these additives are consumed per person per year on average in both foods and medicines. Remember that, while it is compulsory for the ingredients of foods and drinks to be clearly listed, no such legislation exists to protect us where drugs are concerned. The following list of possible additives comes from Dr Richard Mackarness' book, *Chemical Victims*. Bleaches, colours, flavourings, preservatives, thickeners, gums, buffers, acidulants, suspending agents, texture modifiers, emulsifiers, surface-active agents, chelating agents, anti-oxidants, antibacterials, antibiotics, mould retarders, humectants (moisturisers), organic solvents, enzymes, vitamins, minerals, alcohol (eg glycerol, sorbitol and manitol), sweeteners and flavour-potentiators, including sugar, saccharin, dextri-maltose, salt, monosodium glutamate, nucleotides and citric acid.

Why, one wonders, is their use permitted? Nobody wants them. Have you ever met anyone in the supermarket anxiously scanning the list of ingredients muttering 'I must find a brand with more additives'? The general view of those reviewing the research is that toxicology is a very inexact science and that the experiments produce conflicting results and provide insufficient data for true evaluation. As it is known that different species metabolise certain substances quite differently to humans, it seems bad luck on the unfortunate animals to suffer to no avail in the cause of something nobody wants.

On 25 October 1989, the *Daily Telegraph* stated that more than a third of people no longer trust Government assurances that the food they eat is safe. The weekly business magazine *Marketing* said that food scares and contradictory advice on healthy diet have led to confusion. Fewer than one in ten people believe what the Government says on health and safety issues and more than sixty per cent believe the Government glosses over the facts.

In November 1989 the Government proposed some totally inconsistent new controls on food colours (thereby confirming the public's lack of confidence). These were following the ministers' consideration of the Food Advisory Committee's recommendations in its *Review of the Colouring Matter in Food Regulations.* In their report the ministers stated that they now concluded that certain foods should not contain added colouring matter but that in others it is still acceptable. Although the Government opted for 'stricter controls', they stated: 'The responsible use of colours will continue to have a role in providing consumers with a choice of attractively presented foods.' *You* also have a choice – as to whether or not you wish to preserve your future health.

In this Encyclopedia I have listed only those additives which have been shown, through research, to be potentially responsible for each symptom. As allergic and toxic reactions vary in the individual, *do* bear in mind that *any* additive can have an adverse affect on *anyone.*

The Food Additives Campaign Team (FACT) work very hard to protect our food from additives which are known to produce harmful effects on our health. Let us support them in every way we can (see page 202 for their address).

CHAPTER 3

VITAMINS AND MINERALS

The conception, popular amongst orthodox members of the medical profession, that we all get enough vitamins in our diets does not take into account the highly processed foods consumed in large quantities today, the increased amount of vitamins required when people are in poor health or under stress, that heating and cooking destroy many natural vitamins, and that some of us have a much higher requirement than others anyway.

Good health can be maintained, and stress can be minimised, by eating regularly and well, by getting plenty of fresh air and exercise and by getting sufficient sleep. However, more important than all these is that people should be on the right diet. There is only *one* diet, and that is the one which is right for *you*.

In the recommendations in this book for vitamin, mineral and other supplements, I have not quoted specific dosages (with the exception of vitamin C). These need specialist advice, either from a doctor experienced in advising on nutrition, a qualified nutritionist or dietitian or, if self-prescribing, be guided by books such as *Nutritional Medicine* by Dr Stephen Davies and Dr Alan Stewart, or *The Vitamin Bible* by nutritionist Earl Mindell.

People suffering from physical and/or mental symptoms, whether or not there is a relationship with allergies, will benefit from taking supplements. Vitamins A, C and E, and trace minerals zinc and selenium, are especially important for building up immunity.

Vitamin C has antiviral and antibacterial properties and it aids in the healing of wounds. It is the most widely consumed supplement. It is invaluable in minimising the symptoms of colds and other infections. During infections, the vitamin C taken naturally through our diet is depleted and this is the time to increase your intake. Certain drugs, such as antibiotics and aspirin, deplete vitamin C as well. It is a natural antihistamine and will help to prevent and relieve allergic reactions as well as building up the immune system. Vitamin C is needed in the absorption of iron, and so vegetarians would be well advised to take supplements of both. It is said that 25mg of vitamin C is lost with every cigarette. Vitamin C is a powerful anti-oxidant, and high intakes of anti-oxidant vitamins could protect against cancer.

Green leafy vegetables contain anti-oxidant vitamins C and E, and beta-carotene (which is converted in the body to vitamin A.) Beta-carotene is found in carrots, corn, tomatoes, peas, apricots and mangoes, as well as greens, and it could also be a protection against developing cancer.

The B vitamins have been known for years to be good for the nerves. Therefore, whilst they are helpful to all allergy sufferers, they are particularly beneficial to those who suffer from stressful, psychological allergy-induced symptoms. B vitamins should always be taken in a balanced complex unless otherwise prescribed by someone qualified to do so. Vitamins B and C are water-soluble, so the body eliminates what is not required.

Vitamins A, D and E are fat-soluble and are stored in the body so that it is important not to exceed the stated dose. Vitamin A aids in the treatment of many eye disorders. Vitamin D, which is found in fish oils, helps to prevent arthritis and reduces the risk of blood clots. Vitamin E helps to replace the natural oils in one's body and is therefore especially good for women over the age of forty as it helps to keep their skin fresh and supple. It has excellent healing powers when used externally on wounds, burns and other injuries. There is some evidence that it modifies cholesterol and may protect against heart disease. It is found in vegetable oil, nuts, whole grains, green vegetables, milk and eggs.

Many allergic people are found to be low in trace minerals which we all require for good physical and mental health. Those in which we are most likely to be deficient are iron, magnesium, zinc and selenium. If you are anaemic and require iron, the best way to take this is in the form of *Sytron*, which is liquid iron in its natural form with no additives. It can be either prescribed or bought over the counter. Magnesium can be bought on its own or in the form of dolomite, which is magnesium and calcium combined. Those people who cannot tolerate milk and milk products are likely to be low in calcium, and this is a good way in which to take it.

Zinc is recommended by the Hyperactive Children's Support Group which commonly finds hyperactive children to be short of this mineral. Many other allergic people require it too. It has been known for those who lose their sense of taste and smell to recover these faculties after taking a zinc supplement. Many people suffering from mental symptoms are zinc-deficient.

Selenium also seems to benefit allergy sufferers. Selenium and vitamin E are synergistic; this means that they work better together than either would on its own. They are both anti-oxidants, and anti-oxidants are said to slow down the ageing process and protect against developing cancer.

Oil of Evening Primrose has been discovered in recent years to benefit people suffering from premenstrual tension, eczema, hyperactivity, arthritis and other allergies. It contains two essential fatty acids: linoleic and gamma-linoleic acid (GLA); these convert in the body to a substance called prostaglandin E which enhances the immune system and alleviates allergic reactions.

When too many petrochemicals are absorbed into our bodies our digestive enzymes break down and fail to work properly. Restoring the balance of vitamins and minerals helps our digestive enzymes to recover and function as they should.

Some people swear by the benefits of Royal Jelly. It is said to assist in various ailments and to help people reach their own health potential.

It is a milky-white substance which contains minute amounts of a range of B vitamins, amino acids and trace minerals. It may well be that the synergistic effect boosts the immune system to a degree that individual doses of the same ingredients would not. Some brands of supplements are unnecessarily expensive. Others can be bought at much more reasonable prices. One such brand is made by the Cantassium Company whose products are free from all artificial additives and all common food allergens. They can advise on personal requirements. Many children benefit from a strong multi-vitamin and multi-mineral supplement. This needs to be high in B complex vitamins, calcium and iron. Vitamin C will need to be taken separately. Cantassium produces a good additive-free multi-vitamin called *Junamac*. Whatever you buy, make sure it *is* additive-free.

Babies are usually prescribed their own vitamin drops. Just make sure that they contain no colourings or other additives – (they usually don't). Cantassium produces a good multi-vitamin for babies called *Mini-Junamac* which can be given after your baby has been weaned.

The value of all these supplements should never be underestimated as they have played a major role in the recovery of many people whom orthodox medicine has failed to help.

CHAPTER 4

WATER

If you suffer from chronic abdominal pain, diarrhoea or any other symptoms which cannot be related to foods or other allergens, do consider your water supply as the possible villain. Water varies from area to area, and in some places it is still relatively pure. In or near large cities it is more likely to be contaminated, and it will have to have been purified a number of times before it is considered safe for drinking. Small residues in the form of agricultural pollution, industrial discharges and a wide range of chemicals may all be present in our drinking water 'in amounts too small to be considered a danger to health'. Where water is taken from rivers, traces of detergents may also be found. Needless to say, tap water in many areas of the UK does not come up to European standards.

Chlorine is added to all water supplies to control bacteria. There have been extremely few outbreaks of illness caused by bacterial contamination of the water supply. Some people, however, are sensitive to chlorine. In some areas fluoride is added, too; this is said to protect the teeth of young children. Some people are sensitive to this also.

So what about considering a water filter? Would it help, and which one should you choose? *Which* magazine studied this subject in February 1989, and the following are some relevant points which were made.

Manufacturers of jug-type filters claim their filters remove or reduce metals such as lead, copper and zinc as well as water hardness, organic chemicals, chlorine and cloudiness. They don't claim to remove fluoride.

Aluminium occurs naturally in some water supplies and is also used in the purification process. Most, but not all, is removed before it gets into the mains supply (there is growing evidence that aluminium could be associated with Alzheimer's disease). Some jug filters remove aluminium.

Iron and manganese occur naturally in some water supplies, and iron may get in from old pipes. Neither occur in the UK in amounts which make water unsafe to drink. Most jug filters reduce both in hard water.

Lead gets into drinking water mainly from lead pipes found inside some pre-1976 houses or connecting them to the water mains. Large quantities of lead can damage the brain and nervous system, cause anaemia and affect the muscles. The filters tested by the *Which* magazine team were very effective at removing lead, and (they said) these filters should keep levels within safe limits if the filter is changed regularly.

There is much concern about the high level of nitrates in tap water these days. Intensive farming involves a greater use of nitrogen fertilisers. Some of the nitrates get washed into rivers and underground water supplies and eventually find their way into tap water. Only one of the filters which were tested removed nitrates from water, and this was effective only when the filter was fairly new; this is the Waymaster Crystal.

There is concern also regarding organic chemicals used in industry, and all the water filters tested were effective at removing the more common ones from tap water.

The *Which* report stated that the way in which our water supply is organised is likely to change with privatisation. At the time of writing it is supplied by water authorities, or statutory water companies, or it comes direct from private supplies. Whoever you pay for your water is responsible for maintaining its quality. All water intended for drinking should meet standards laid down in an EC Directive but some supplies do not. Environmental Health Officers are responsible for checking the quality of all water supplies. The Government aims to see that most of these private supplies meet EC standards by 1995.

Which states: 'Water authorities and statutory water companies say they will investigate any complaints. They will also tell you what is in your water and give advice. Most will visit your house, take samples and analyse your water, sometimes free of charge. If your water comes from a private supply it may be less easy to get complaints investigated. Many authorities will inspect your plumbing and check the amount of lead in your tap water free of charge. If your pipes are in poor condition, you may be able to get a grant from your local council to help with the cost. All suppliers of water have a legal duty to supply "wholesome" water, so if you are unhappy with your water and the action taken by your local supplier, refer your complaint to your local Environmental Health Officer'.

The water filters investigated in the report were Addis Filtaware, Brita 'fill and pour', Leifheit Aquapur, Habitat, Waterboy and Waymaster Crystal, of which they said: 'Overall the filters were fairly successful at tackling the problems. All the filters removed lead, trichloroethylene and polycyclic aromatic hydrocarbons from both hard and soft water, and iron and manganese from hard but not soft. Only the Waymaster Crystal reduced the amount of nitrates'. They went on to say that a jug filter won't improve the *taste* of water. Their best buys were the Waymaster Crystal or the Boots' Water Filter sold at around the same price.

The *Which* report gave four tips for using a jug filter; these were:
1. Always follow the manufacture's instructions, particularly about when to change the cartridge; keeping a record of the amount you have filtered will help.
2. Don't leave filtered, or indeed any, water standing around for several days; that is what leads to bacterial growth.
3. Keep filtered water in a fridge.
4. Give the water reservoir and jug a weekly clean.

The manufacturers of the filters point out that filtered water, like tap water, should be boiled if it is to be used in baby food.

With regard to bottled water, their recommended best buys for sparkling water were Ashbourne and Sainsbury's Scottish Spring. Their recommended best buys for still were Chiltern Hills, Evian, Glendale Spring, Safeway Braenisge Spring, Tesco Mountain Spring and Volvic.

CHAPTER 5

ELIMINATION AND CANDIDA DIETS

What we eat and drink have a strong influence on our health – present and future. A balanced diet of pure, fresh, natural foods is the ideal and, unless we have a sensitivity to something, can do us only good.

People who reject natural foods in preference to instant, processed, artificial-additive-containing foods are undoubtedly jeopardising their future health. We all want quick meals occasionally so, when you do, go for the canned, packaged or frozen foods which are relatively *free from artificial additives*. Plenty exist if you look for them, and after a while it will become second nature.

Allergic people produce too much acid, but this is not necessarily a result of taking too many acidic foods. There are more people, for instance, unable to tolerate cow's milk than any other so-called natural product. Cow's milk is alkaline – the converse of acidic – and yet this produces acid in many of those who are sensitive to it! That many people do react to it is not surprising as it contains a foreign protein (one intended for consumption by calves, not humans) and, due to man's own efforts, traces of antibiotics and hormones as well. Taking a glass of warm water with a teaspoonful of sodium bicarbonate helps to counteract the inevitable build-up of acid in allergic people. That 'Monday morning feeling' or, indeed, a hangover for whatever reason will be more hastily dispersed by this method also but should not be used continually.

So what is the purpose of an elimination diet? It is the only means by which an individual can discover for himself which foods he is allergic to without recourse to the services of a doctor.

The foods chosen for use on the elimination are those which are least likely to cause allergy symptoms; those which are *most* likely to be causing your symptoms have been excluded. The diet must be taken for as long as it takes for the symptoms to clear (or at least show signs of clearing). In most cases this will be under a week. A few people may take slightly longer, even up to two weeks, but I do not recommend continuing the diet for longer than that. If you notice no improvement but still feel that your problems are due to allergies, it may be that you are one of a very small minority who are allergic to one of the foods on the diet. The other possibility is that you are suffering from an overriding inhalant allergy to something at home or in your place of work. Going away for a few days could help to clarify this point.

Some people suffer from masked allergies, which are really the same as delayed reactions. You may even feel better temporarily after taking certain foods or drinks (as with alcohol for the alcoholic). This boost-up may last for several hours before you relapse into your chronically unwell condition. You may return to the offending food again without realising that this is a subconscious reaction carried out in order to feel better, thereby setting the cycle in motion again. If you find that you are craving a particular food or drink, you are likely to be allergic to it.

To return to the elimination diet, it is important for you to know that, in *some* cases, withdrawal symptoms may be experienced. They can take any form, but headaches and other aches and pains are the most likely. Coffee and tea withdrawals are common, but this can apply equally to any food or drink. If you already have a good idea what you are sensitive to you can either withdraw gradually (ie make each cup of coffee or tea slightly weaker than the last) or you can take your usual medication over the first few days to cover you (bearing in mind that medicines can also be a source of allergen!).

No one should cut out any medication prescribed by their doctor without his consent. However, it must not be forgotten that many drugs can cause side-effects. These are often caused not so much by the drugs themselves but by a variety of additives used as colourings, flavourings, binders etc. Coming off tranquillizers is an important part of recovery in this illness. Hopefully, the patient will lose the need for them after allergens have been discovered and eliminated and confidence has been regained.

Not everyone suffers from withdrawals, but if you do, at least you have the satisfaction of knowing that you are definitely on the right track! These symptoms, in the majority of people, should have started to clear by the fourth or fifth day when you will notice a marked improvement. (A smaller number of people will take longer than a week, and a few may even take up to two weeks.) An elimination diet is easy to prescribe. Actually going on to one takes willpower. Where children are concerned, the idea of a diet is greatly enhanced by the use of 'star charts' for co-operation and the incentive of a reward at the end. The elimination diets given here are equally suitable for children.

Everyone going on to an elimination diet can take as much of the foods allowed as often as they wish. In fact, you are recommended to eat or drink something every two to three hours. It is advisable to keep a record of all foods and drinks taken and any reactions experienced when re-introducing new foods.

The elimination diet consists of lamb, chicken, turkey, cod, plaice, haddock, cabbage, courgettes, leeks, carrots, celery, swede, turnip, parsnips, pears, peaches, plums, apricots, brown rice, sea salt (buy sea salt without the pouring agent sodium hexacyanoferrate II), bottled water and rice cakes. (The latter are obtainable from health food shops.)

For those people who are not positively *ill*, who do not have *very* severe symptoms, or who feel that they simply cannot face such a meagre diet, I suggest adding the following: dried apricots (dried apricots should be bought [from health food shops] without sulphur dioxide), raisins, unsweetened soya milk, clear honey, ground rice, salad and other vegetables (excluding peas and beans) and other fruits (excluding citrus fruits). (Even with these additional foods you will still be excluding the most common food allergens which include wheat, gluten (found in wheat, oats, barley and rye), cow's milk, eggs, beef, pork, sugar, chocolate, cheese, yeast, alcohol, tea, coffee and all chemical additives).

All these foods should be taken in their natural form with nothing added, and they can be boiled, steamed, grilled or oven-baked. Vegetables must be cooked in bottled water only. Remember, you can eat as much as you wish as often as you like. Here is a suggested menu for those people who decide to include the additional foods.

BREAKFAST

Ground rice cooked with soya milk and served with honey. Banana or other fruit. Rice cakes with honey (no butter or margarine). Bottled water to drink.

PACKED LUNCH

Rice cakes with cold lamb, chicken or turkey, and any salad you wish (no butter or margarine). Dried apricots, raisins, bananas and/or other fruit. Cooked rice with raisins, peppers, carrots, onions and sea salt (remember to take a spoon for this). Bottled water to drink.

EVENING MEAL

Cooked lamb, chicken or turkey, cod, plaice or haddock served with rice and as many vegetables as you wish. Fruit for afters. Bottled water to drink. Alternatively, serve cold meat with rice and salad.

SNACKS

You can snack on anything so far listed. For extra warmth and nutrition boil up any meat bones or carcasses for stock using bottled water only. Add vegetables and simmer until tender. Season with sea salt.

When your symptoms have cleared you can start re-testing. I suggest that you test your tap water first. If you experience a reaction then continue with bottled water for the time being (for cooking also). Later you can buy a water purifier. When re-testing foods, test only one at a time and try only very small quantities to start with to avoid any bad reactions. If in doubt you can try a larger quantity next time. It is simpler to test only one food in twenty-four hours as some reactions may be delayed. Even those which are delayed for a number of hours can cause severe allergic reactions. It is people who suffer from intolerances for whom it is the most complicated. Whereas an *allergy* can produce a positive and possibly severe reaction after only one ingestion, you may need to take a large quantity or consume a food for several consecutive days before an *intolerance* manifests itself. The only clue I can give you is to say that among the foods most commonly causing intolerance (or allergy) are cow's milk, wheat, gluten (in wheat, oats, barley and rye), eggs and yeast. Try giving each one up in turn for a week and see whether you feel better for it.

When you experience a reaction wait until you are symptom-free before testing the next food. This will take a little time but is well worth persevering with in order to avoid confusion.

If you have been able to make use of the information you have read so far, you will know that the well-known phrase 'you are what you eat' applies to you. The extent of your recovery depends on the degree to which you are affected and your ability and determination to avoid those things which make you ill, although, of course, there are many other interrelated factors. It is, for instance, very important to be particularly careful with your diet after a stressful experience, such as having 'flu, which lowers your immune system, making you temporarily more sensitive. After discovering and eliminating your worst allergens, and when you have remained well for some time, you will find that some previous allergens can be better tolerated because you have raised your allergy threshold.

If you are a multiple allergy sufferer, it is advisable to rotate your foods from now on so that you avoid eating the same foods every day. Doctors often advise a four day rotation diet (eating different foods each day for four days and then starting again). This precaution is worth following as far as possible becauses it minimises the chances of developing new allergies.

For those few unfortunate people who appear to be allergic to *every-thing*, I suggest excluding the very *worst* foods and giving yourself a diet of a small amount of a wide variety of mixed foods at every meal time. In this manner you will never feel a hundred per cent, I know, but you will avoid any really *severe* reactions and it will also ensure that you are getting the necessary nuitrients.

Candida albicans is a common yeast which we all have in our gut as part of the natural intestinal flora. When there is an overgrowth of the wrong kind of gut flora this causes a condition known as candidiasis – a problem which is on the increase. The reason for this is said to be due to the extensive use of antibiotics, the Pill, and an increased sugar consumption. In the medical profession there is some controversy as to just how widespread this is. Certain doctors and alternative therapists are very keen on putting their patients on a 'candida' diet; thus, some people who subsequently turn out to be allergic to food or chemicals are put on a candida diet unnecessarily. Of course, you *can* suffer from both. The most commonly reported symptoms of candidiasis are diarrhoea, wind, abdominal pain and bloating. (These are also common gut allergy symptoms.) Candidiasis can be accompanied by other symptoms and is more likely in someone who already suffers from thrush (candidiasis of mouth, vagina, penis or skin). To be successful, the candida diet must be taken over a period of months. The purpose of the diet is to avoid all those foods which promote the growth of the 'bad' gut flora. These are sugars, yeast, wheat, oats, rye, most fresh fruits, dried fruits, mushrooms, cheese, nuts, seeds and spices. The foods recommended for a candida diet are as follows: rice flour, potato flour, soya flour, chick pea flour, any and all vegetables, potatoes, rice, soya and olive oils, sunflower and safflower oils, butter, chicken, duck, turkey, beef, lamb, pork, rabbit, eggs, shellfish, all fresh and tinned fish, split peas, chick peas, rhubarb, melon, soya milk and tomato juice. When advocating this diet, doctors normally prescribe an antifungal agent such as nystatin. Capricin is another alternative, and can be bought at health food shops without prescription. For the most effective result the diet and an antifungal agent should be used in conjunction.

CHAPTER 6

YOUR ENVIRONMENT

People with allergic tendencies have to be constantly aware of their environment. Sensitivity to climate must also be taken into account. Everyone differs, and their ability to tolerate climatic changes differs too. By the sea, or up a mountain on a fine, clear day is about the safest and healthiest of all atmospheres. Avoid cold climates and strong winds if these affect you, and damp climates are best avoided by everyone – especially those with asthmatic, bronchial or arthritic problems. The majority of allergy sufferers will be better in warm, sunny climes and some people who have a dry, eczematous skin will find that it clears completely in warm sunshine. A few people are sun-sensitive and this may be a side-effect of a drug they are, or have been, taking.

POLLEN

It will be necessary for some people to watch out for the various pollen seasons. Trees produce pollen in March, April and May, and the grass pollen season is June and July. Flowers pollinate throughout the summer, and one of the most allergenic is the chrysanthemum – which appears in late summer. Moulds cause allergies in the autumn, and mould growths can gather in air conditioners during the winter months and can affect people when air conditioners are turned on again.

MOVING HOUSE

Sometimes people are so allergic to their present environment that they feel it advisable to move house in the hope of improving their health. This must be given careful consideration in order not to exchange one set of problems for another. The following comments are worth some thought, although it would probably be impracticable to try to follow them all.

Try to live at least five miles away from any factory to avoid atmospheric pollutants.

Whenever possible, avoid a house near main roads with parking meters because of excessive exhaust fumes.

Do not live too near any fields because of the dangers of grass pollen and the chemical fertilisers and pesticides which may be used.

Avoid a house with large trees in the garden or near by, especially pine trees which are a known source of allergen to some people.

People with breathing problems particularly should try to avoid low-lying land or a house near water because of dampness.

If necessary, avoid a house with gas fires. Anyone who already knows he is gas-allergic will need an all-electric house.

Do not buy a house with cavity wall insulation, or floors which require polishing because of the high allergenic properties of the chemicals involved.

Avoid a house near a nursery garden or any place where spraying may be done, because the droplets of the chemicals involved will be airborne.

An allergic person is better off in a south- or west-facing bedroom as dampness and cold rooms can lead to asthma and bronchitis. If you should be so unfortunate as to discover that the house you bought has a tendency to damp, then a strong light bulb should give out enough heat in a small room (if kept on constantly) to prevent dampness accumulating. Similarly, a light bulb in a clothes or shoe cupboard will stop the contents from going mouldy.

When planning the layout of your rooms remember that indoor plants, especially those with hairy leaves – such as primulas – can cause rashes, runny nose, swelling around the eyes etc.

HOLIDAYS

Food Allergy Sufferers

The best thing you can do before going off on holiday is to ask your doctor to prescribe you some Nalcrom (sodium cromoglycate). This is a food allergy blocker which works well for most people. Few people suffer side-effects, but those who react to beef will need to remove the gelatin casing and take only the powder. The orthodox way to prescribe it is to recommend two capsules four times a day. This gives general coverage. However, those people who *know* what they are allergic to may choose to eat only 'safe' foods during the day and save their Nalcrom for the evening meal. Four capsules taken from a quarter of an hour up to one hour before the meal will be their most effective way to use Nalcrom.

Check with the manager when booking into a hotel that he has a sympathetic attitude to people on special diets. I have always found this to be so but it is far better to make your position clear *before* you arrive. After your arrival it is advisable to check before *each* meal in order to avoid any mistakes. Do not risk any compound foods if your reactions could be severe or prolonged. Rather than a pudding, for example, it is better to stick to a simple piece of fruit and play safe. If all this is too much to contemplate, you are better off going self-catering.

Chemical Allergy Sufferers

It is advisable to check when booking that the hotel you intend visiting is set well away from factories, busy main roads, etc. If you suffer from tree, flower or grass pollens, do check that you are going out of season or, at least, will be well removed from them.

Check when booking that the hotel (and especially your bedroom) has not been painted recently and that it is not placed directly over the kitchen or any gas or oil-fired boilers or other source of outlet for fumes. Check also that they do not have polished floors or use furniture polish in the bedrooms (or at least in yours). See whether there is a non-smoking area in the public rooms. If you are allergic to feathers, wool or polyester, you will have to check on what type of bedding they use. One of your major problems may be other people's perfume. You will just have to be thick-skinned and ask to move your table if it should become necessary. Avoid very old hotels or those in low-lying areas which are more likely to be damp.

Chemical Victims member Betty Hardcastle can provide you with a list of accommodation catering for the needs of allergy sufferers. Her address is at the back of the book.

CASE HISTORY

I did not plan to include any case histories as such, as these are covered under the heading 'Research'. However, when I received this first-hand detailed series of events, I was so impressed at the lengths to which someone would go to see justice done that I asked permission to include it in this book.

The gentleman concerned is, by profession, a chemist. He has, therefore, an intimate knowledge of the chemicals which he and his family have had to endure. As a chemist he must also have had some standing in the eyes of those people whose support he sought. Yet not one agreed to help him. Was this a case of 'not wanting to get involved', was it cowardice, or was it plain ignorance? You can judge for yourselves.

On 14 September 1989, my wife, Mary, contacted our local Environmental Health Department complaining of the emissions of chemicals from the vent of a small workshop at the back of our next door neighbours. We had tried to be very reasonable with the occupier and had told him that the emission from his spraying process was making us very drowsy and giving us head-aches, together with physical and mental fatigue, pains in the chest and various other symptoms. I had taken Mary and my son, John, to see him on various occasions to show him the effects this was having upon them.

He apologised and said he would remove the vent to a very high position which would, together with the installation of a water filter, hopefully eliminate the emission of the solvent. But he did not do anything. As we were were not getting anywhere with him privately, we put our hopes in the Environmental Health Department. We thought they would stop the process altogether. We had not contacted them earlier because we did not like to put him out of work.

Unfortunately, after the investigation, the Environmental Health

Department could not substantiate our complaint. They said they were totally satisfied with his operation and they recommended a new location for the vent where the opening is in line with the ridge of the roof. A water filter was not mentioned. It was to my horror to see this happening. It will certainly affect a number of people over a larger area after a period of time, especially the residents opposite who are now in the 'firing line' of the emissions.

Since September our health has gradually deteriorated and the symptoms have occurred more frequently and with greater intensity. This has spurred us on to request help from various departments, consultants and university research units. From the information I have collated I realise that my family has been suffering from what is known in America as 'chemical induced immune system dysfunction'. In other words, chemical overload of the immune system. As a result of this we have become very sensitive to common chemicals and many foods.

Since October we have requested help from the Prime Minister, our Member of Parliament, the Health and Safety Executive, the Department of the Environment, the Health and Safety Commission, Occupational Health Consultants from various universities, the European Commission, the Royal Society of Chemistry, the World Health Organisation, HM Pollution Control and various private consultants including six top allergy experts but nobody wanted to get involved with the dispute.

Based on the report by the County Analyst (who monitored the emissions on 7 November 1989) the Environmental Health Department claims that the level of the emission from the vent offers no health hazard to the residents. I, as a qualified chemist, have pointed out to them on numerous occasions that the report was totally unprofessional, inadequate and inconclusive. At the same time, I have passed on to them much literature detailing the hazardous effects of solvents on human health. Also I have given them the names of consultants to contact. However, the Head of the Environmental Health Department said it was not justifiable to spend more than £200 on an investigation for just one family. (He consistently chose to disregard the other sufferers, calling their illness 'circumstantial'.)

The report is hardly acceptable as our neighbour was observed for one week only during which he naturally co-operated with the authorities. Since then this report has been used by all the various departments and regulating bodies contacted. Nobody within these departments has studied the validity of it. It is the unquestioning acceptance of the report which has created much of our suffering and prolonged our agony.

It was in November 1989, when our physical health and mental ability had deteriorated to such a frightening extent, that we were faced with no other choice but to leave our home and close our business where we had lived and worked since 1982. Had we accepted this report and our GP's advice, as did all the authorities we contacted at this time, we would all be dead by now or have ended up in a mental home.

I have strong evidence to prove that the test carried out by the County Analyst for this purpose was totally meaningless. I have a number of independent witnesses and fellow-sufferers as a result of exposure to these emissions. I also have good reason to believe that EHD and the HSE have not carried out their investigations thoroughly with adequate attention to detail. Although we have seen our GP on various occasions, we found it necessary to arrange for ourselves admission to the Breakspear Hospital to have intensive tests and treatment by experts. The costs so far amount to over £30,000.

Evidence of the nature of the emissions, proof of the inadequacy of the County Analyst's test, evidence from witnesses and various other forms of evidence are available for inspection.

The relationship between our illness and the emission is under research. There are legal difficulties as it is a new area of study. The Health and Safety Executive is only interested in statutory safety limits and totally ignores the effect on our immunity of multiple chemical exposure even at low concentration levels. That is why so many people in the past have had to give up their pursuit of justice as everybody will advise them that, at the end of the day, there will not be sufficient proof to satisfy a court of law.

I believe these solvent emissions were a contributory factor in the death of my mother-in-law in July 1989. Her bedroom was only a few yards away from the opening of the vent.

July 1990. In the past six months I have conducted a questionnaire and have found almost a hundred people in the surrounding area suffering from common symptoms of toxic exposure. These are asthma, skin rashes, coughs and 'flu-like symptoms, headache, sore throat, tight chest, catarrh, nasal blockage, pins and needles, confusion, depression, loss of appetite, tiredness, lack of concentration, weakness of limbs, fatigue after eating, sore eyes, painful joints, aggressiveness, intoxication after very small amounts of alcohol, hangover headaches unrelated to alcohol, muscular tremor, muscle twitching, inability to move limbs, increasing arthritic pains, sensitive teeth, bleeding gums, painful and heavy periods, creaking joints, earache, excessively sweaty feet, loss of taste, painful neck, diarrhoea, and an increasing loss of strength in the little finger. Hair loss is increasing in women and children as well as men, and dandruff and skin changes are apparent.

Our friend, a man of quite exceptional tenacity and enterprise, will not give up his quest for justice. He will not hesitate to take whatever steps he feels necessary to protect his family and neighbours from the effects of toxic pollution being constantly expelled into their environment, a process which, at this moment in time, is legally totally acceptable.

December 1990. I am delighted to report that I have just learned that at last support is being offered by people in high places. It will be a long-drawn-out battle, but it just goes to show that tenacity and determination pay off!

CHAPTER 7

DOCTORS

I was lucky enough to have a doctor who made the original diagnosis of my allergies some twenty years ago – a fact I have now come to regard as remarkable. So it is with no personal bitterness, but only through the experience of others, that I say it seems extraordinary that so many doctors are still unable to accept the growing incidence of food and chemical allergies. This is in spite of scientific research being frequently published in well-known medical journals.

One of the ironies, therefore, of allergy-induced illness is that many people suffer not only the discomfort of the symptoms but insults from the medical profession as well. I will give you some examples of the responses received by people from their doctors or the specialists to whom they have been referred: that they are imagining their symptoms; that there is nothing wrong with them; that such symptoms are to be expected at their age; that they are suffering from stress; that they have brought their problems upon themselves; that they are over-anxious; that their marital problems are to blame; that they are neurotic, or that they simply like to visit their doctor! Some of the comments made to mothers of allergic children are even more weird: that the child is faking his symptoms to gain attention; that his symptoms are due to *her* marital problems; that her (thin) child is probably anorexic; that her (fat) child steals food; that he is just plain naughty; that she (the mother) is jumping on the allergy bandwagon; that she is over-anxious, over-protective or domineering, or that she imagines her child suffers from allergies because she does herself. Whether the ignorance of these doctors surpasses their arrogance or vice versa is debatable. What is not in doubt is that they cause a great deal of distress. In fact there may be many who are not willing to concede publicly what they secretly believe to be true because they have not the courage to do so. There is evidence, however, that an increasing number of doctors are coming down off the fence because they have seen the facts staring them in the face. Those are the ones who observe and listen. A doctor who is prepared to learn something from his patient must be a good doctor. If you have a good doctor who admits he knows little on this subject, or a bad doctor who is not interested, what do you do? You need to contact an allergy association. They can give you information which will enable you to make great strides in correcting your problems yourself, or, if you prefer it, give you names of doctors working in the field of allergy and environmental illness. Even amongst these doctors you will have to be careful. Some use unscientific forms of testing and treatment, and others take only diet into consideration and ignore the fact that this should be done in conjunction with the consideration of inhalant allergies to be properly valid. Beware of anyone (doctor or otherwise) who offers hair testing to diagnose allergies – this is of no scientific value whatsoever. (It *can* be used to test the balance of trace minerals in the body when done under properly controlled scientific conditions.)

So, you may well ask, what doctor and/or treatment can I have confidence in? I should say straight away that, unless you are covered by medical insurance (BUPA and PPP cover this area but not all insurance companies do), outpatient treatment will cost you hundreds of pounds and in-patient treatment will run into thousands. Experienced doctors who take patients on the NHS *outside* their own area are very few and far between and would certainly have long waiting lists.

However, if you still wish to go ahead, my advice is that you look for a doctor with several years experience practising either enzyme-potentiated desensitisation (EPD) or intradermal testing and neutralisation. The allergy associations can discuss the benefits of these treatments with you. They can also give you lots of help themselves, so if you cannot afford the fees, do not despair; help and advice are at hand.

EPD was first developed by Dr Len McEwen in 1966. Since then it has become a much more sophisticated vaccine which contains a wide range of common foods and some of the more commonly inhaled allergens. The principle behind this treatment is that you will be given a general desensitisation to cover all the things to which you *may* be intolerant. This might involve some initial adverse reactions but you should improve over a period of time, thus requiring less frequent doses. On average, people stabilise their allergies on a maintenance dose of twice a year.

Intradermal testing is a form of testing whereby each food or inhalant is tested individually by injection over a range of strengths to ascertain at which point the patient reacts. Sublingual drops can then be made up for each food or chemical so that the patient can desensitise himself daily, thereby tolerating the allergen with no ill-effect. Drops can be re-ordered, but neutralising points may change over a period of time and the tests will then need to be carried out again.

Doctors may also use elimination diets instead of, or as well as, other forms of testing and treatment. Although no treatment can ever be found to suit everyone, I am in no doubt from the reports I have received over the years that both enzyme-potentiated desensitisation and intradermal testing and neutralisation have helped a great many people return to good health.

In conclusion, I believe that people should be made aware of the workings of their own bodies and take more responsibility for their health upon themselves. Many already so do and, of course, there are others who, for one reason or another, are unable to do this; however, even the least able have some observations to offer which a wise doctor will take into account. If doctor and patient could work as a team, combining the doctor's experience and expertise with the patient's self-awareness, this would not only lead to a healthier population but considerably ease the doctor's case load as well!

So what is our hope for the future? In America, allergists can pass examinations set by the Board of Allergy and Immunology. No similar opportunity exists in Britain. However, there are signs that more than one eminent consultant is taking steps to ensure that training posts will be created in order that new medical students and existing doctors may be taught about environmentally induced illness. Not before time! I believe that the day will come when to say that you do not believe in food and chemical allergies will cause as much mirth as to say that you do not believe in the germ theory.

CHAPTER 8

DRUGS AND ANAESTHETICS

Any of the symptoms referred to under individual headings in this book are as likely to be caused by the side-effects of drugs as anything else. These will not *necessarily* be those which are anticipated by the manufacturers, as individual allergic reactions may be experienced. In the case of tranquillisers, the side-effects may continue for some considerable time after you have stopped taking them. It may be that they alter the immune system which could account for the side-effects being prolonged long after the drug is stopped. In any case, coming off tranquillisers is an important part of recovery in allergic illness. All this should be taken into consideration before going through the motions of an elimination diet. If you believe a drug you are taking is causing side-effects, then discuss this with your doctor. There are always other options.

A wide variety of pills and medicines contain colourings and preservatives which can cause urticaria, asthma and other allergic reactions. White tablets are usually free from these additives so they are preferable. Boots the Chemist do a range of children's medicines which are free from artificial colourings. Caffeine is present in many over-the-counter tonics and pain relievers, such as Anadin. There is no legal requirement to specify ingredients but these can be investigated by your chemist if necessary. Unfortunately, though, pharmaceutical companies tell neither chemists nor anyone else when they decide to change the composition of their drugs.

Taking the Pill, which is a steroid, can make women more susceptible to developing allergies than they otherwise would be. Younger women are especially likely to develop serious chemical imbalances leading to multiple allergies and long-term reproductive difficulties. Certain drugs can affect our vitamin and mineral balance. Long-term use of corticosteroids has been found to be related to lower zinc levels. Also, this will produce many undesirable side-effects but long-term use of *low*-dose corticosteroids or short-term use can be helpful in certain forms of allergic disease. Long-term use of aspirin leads to a deficiency of vitamin C and folic acid. Lack of folic acid can cause anaemia and digestive disturbances.

Prolonged use of antibiotics can induce allergic reactions and candidiasis and should be avoided whenever there is an alternative. However, if you have been prescribed antibiotics, it is very important to complete the course, unless you should develop an allergic reaction, in which case you must inform your doctor. A number of people are allergic to penicillin. It is possible that such people may not be able to tolerate milk and/or beef either because most cows are fed a maintenance dose of antibiotics.

When you need to take an antihistamine for an unavoidable allergen, such as a seasonal one, it is worth gradually cutting down on the prescribed dose to find the smallest amount which will suffice. If you suffer from symptoms which could be dangerous, such as asthma, do not do this without discussing it with your doctor. Nor should you cut down on any other drugs without medical supervision. *Hismanal* and *Triludan* are amongst the best choice of antihistamines for adults as they do not cause the side-effect of drowsiness. Antihistamines for children are as follows:

Phenergan – a syrup which is produced by May and Baker Pharmaceuticals Ltd, is recommended for children from one year upwards. It contains the colour caramel and the preservatives sodium sulphite, sodium metabisulphite and sodium benzoate.

Triludan syrup, made by Merrell Dow Pharmaceuticals is suitable for 6–12 year olds. It contains artificial sweeteners lycasin and saccharin, preservative benzyl alcohol and banana flavouring. It does not contain any colourings.

Piriton syrup, made by Allen and Hanburys, can be given to children aged 1–12 years (discuss suitable dosage with your pharmacist or doctor). It contains standard syrup preparations; the preservative is a mixture of hydroxybenzoates. It is flavoured with tingle flavour and contains no colouring agents.

All these drugs are widely used and play a valuable role in helping to relieve the symptoms of allergic children. However, certain additives may affect some children, so you will need to watch out for this. Adding preservatives to medicines is almost unavoidable in the interests of safety. The only exception to this is in *extreme* medical circumstances when a doctor can approach the manufacturer for a preservative-free version of an antihistamine. This would need to be made up on a daily basis to prevent the growth of bacteria.

People who are intolerant of many drugs may be low in the enzyme glutathione peroxidase, which is required in the metabolism of drugs and chemicals. This enzyme requires selenium for its activity. After taking this supplement for a month or two you may find that you are better able to tolerate drugs. You can have a blood test for this at Biolab in London. (You will not find the option available at your local hospital.)

Allergy sufferers are in great need of the pharmaceutical industry to develop new drugs to block and reverse the mechanism of allergic reactions rather than merely reduce the symptoms. In the meantime, one of our best allergy-blocking drugs is sodium cromoglycate (sometimes known as disodium cromoglycate) which comes in the form of *Nalcrom* as a food-allergy blocker, *Intal* for asthmatics, *Rynacrom* for rhinitis and *Opticrom* for eye allergies. It is not absorbed into the blood stream, suits most people, and is known for its safety record.

Medicines : a Guide for Everybody is an excellent book written by Professor Peter Parish. It is regularly updated and well worth buying. Professor Parish has dedicated himself to encouraging the safe and appropriate use of medicines. He has had a distinguished career as a family doctor and researcher and believes that many adverse effects of drugs could be avoided with proper communication between doctor, pharmacist and patient. He has provided information about drugs for the lay person whom he feels is entitled to know what he is being prescribed, and why, and is also entitled to be warned of any dangers relating to each drug.

Another option is to go to your local reference library and ask for *Martindale's Pharmacopoeia* – in which you will be able to look up all available information relating to any particular drug.

It is perhaps a little unusual to publish promotional material in a book but I felt that every allergy sufferer has a right to know what is the situation regarding anaesthetics. I know that adverse reactions to anaesthetics are high on the list of fears of allergy sufferers. Therefore, I am grateful to the Diagnostics Division of Pharmacia Limited who, through Ledger Bennett PR Ltd, have given their permission for the following information to be included in this book. It was sent to me in August 1990. Until then, I had not known of the existence of the National Adverse Anaesthetic Reaction Advisory Service (NAARAS) and the valuable service they offer.

This same information has also been sent to all MPs with an interest in health, to the Chief Medical Officer Sir Donald Acheson and to members of the National Health Bill standing committee.

INCIDENCE OF FATAL REACTIONS TO COMMONLY USED ANAESTHETIC DRUGS

Every year, 3.5 million operations are carried out in the UK under general anaesthesia. Drugs such as suxamethonium and thiopentone are used in over 60 per cent of such operations.

According to the National Adverse Anaesthetic Reaction Advisory Service (NAARAS), Royal Hallamshire Hospital, Sheffield, 5,000 to 10,000 patients per annum suffer an adverse reaction to commonly used anaesthetic drugs such as suxamethonium, thiopentone and alcuronium. Severe reactions occur in perhaps 300 to 500 patients per annum, with effects varying from death to (perhaps even more devastating for the family) severe brain damage.

NAARAS has offered a severe reaction advisory service to anaesthetists for fifteen years and does not solicit work – anaesthetists use the service by choice, and by doing so they indicate that the problem is very real. From 1 January to 27 December 1989, NAARAS has investigated 169 adverse reactions, including four deaths. These numbers are the tip of the iceberg, as only very serious cases are forwarded for investigation.

The cost to the family of a patient who suffers death or severe brain damage cannot be quantified.

Until very recently, laboratory tests to diagnose patients at risk of suffering an adverse reaction have not been available. However, very recently the Diagnostics Division of Pharmacia Limited – a Swedish health care company with a UK base in Milton Keynes – has developed diagnostic tests for sensitivity to anaesthetic agents which have been assessed by Dr E. S. K. Assem, Department of Pharmacology, University College, London (also Honorary Consultant Physician at University College and Middlesex Hospitals, London).

Pharmacia is recognised as the world leader in the field of allergy testing, and has for many years supplied hospitals and laboratories with tests for a variety of allergies – including the more common pollen, animal fur, house-dust mite, foods and penicillin. Using the same well-trusted technology, Pharmacia has developed test kits for suxamethonium, thiopentone and alcuronium.

Aberdeen area health authority has taken the lead, and the local allergy laboratory now offers a routine service to anaesthetists. This was in response to a fatal accident enquiry (8/9 May 1989) into the tragic death of a young mother who was admitted for a routine sterilisation operation in 1987. Sadly, the woman died two days after administration of the anaesthetic drugs thiopentone and suxamethonium without gaining consciousness. Tests carried out at the Sheffield laboratory of NAARAS showed the presence of antibodies to the drug suxamethonium in her blood.

Press releases have been recently sent out announcing the availability of these new test kits to the laboratory and medical press as well as to Sunday, national and local newspapers, TV and radio.

'Medicine Now', broadcast by Radio 4, recently featured the problem of adverse reactions to anaesthetics, and Dr John Watkins, director of NAARAS, spoke on the programme. The response from the public is still coming in (19 August 1990) via telephone calls and letters; although the numbers may be considered small they indicate that this problem is real and that patients are experiencing a lack of information from their anaesthetist about their condition and ways to overcome the problem.

Whilst Dr Watkins and Dr Assem do not advocate full-scale screening, it seems reasonable that patients who have had an adverse reaction should be tested and that allergies of this nature are discussed fully with the patient so that, in the absence of notes, there may be a good chance that the patient can give the doctor this important and relevant information when requested.

The Association of Anaesthetists of Great Britain and Ireland has recently stated that a working party has been set up to consider the matter raised by the tragic death of Mrs Ann McNeill (8/9 May 1989) –

namely, the detection of the risk of anaphylaxis from anaesthetic drugs. Dr Assem has been invited by the Association of Anaesthetists to participate in this working party.

The response so far obtained from patients indicates that they would like to be able to be tested – if not on the NHS then many would gladly pay around £38.00 for peace of mind. At the moment Dr Watkins and Dr Assem can test only those patients who are referred to them by GPs or anaesthetists.

For further information please contact Ann Faulkner, Ledger Bennett PR Limited, Haywood House, Lake Street, Leighton Buzzard, Bedfordshire LU7 8RS, England (tel [0525] 383883).

CHAPTER 9

SELF HELP

If you suffer from chronic or recurring symptoms for which your doctor is unable to give you a diagnosis, you may wish to ask for a second opinion. You are absolutely within your rights to do so, although he is not obliged to send you to the doctor of your choice. Most clinical ecologists request a letter of referral these days so it is to be hoped that your doctor will be agreeable to refer you to one, because they will be looking for causes whereas most other medical people will simply be treating the symptoms. However, unless you are covered by medical insurance, you are likely to be faced with exorbitant medical fees.

So how about doing what you can to help yourself? You have already decided you may be sensitive to something you are eating or inhaling. What do you need to do about it? There are three golden rules : look to your diet, clean up your environment and build up your immunity. You are aiming at controlling your body instead of your body controlling you!

DIET

For a start you can cut out all the artificial additives in your diet (see Chapter 2). Going on to a diet of pure, fresh, wholesome foods may be all you need to rid yourself of a build-up of toxins and feel well again. If you have not lost all your symptoms after this then you must consider going on to an elimination diet (see Chapter 5). This should turn up something, and your next stage is to eliminate the offending foods and/or drinks and look for substitutes. A visit to your health food shop will give you new ideas. Don't be afraid to ask for suggestions. I am sure they will be pleased to advise you.

ENVIRONMENT

With regard to cleaning up your environment, read the introduction and ask yourself the questions listed there. Have you removed all scented toiletries and scented household cleaning materials and replaced them with unscented ones? These are the major hazards in your home, especially when they come in aerosols or sprays. You don't need a special brand of window cleaner – vinegar will do just as well. You don't need a scented furniture polish – use beeswax instead. There are always substitutes for everything. Air fresheners contain formaldehyde – get rid of them!

Boots the Chemist does PVC gloves for those who suffer from a rubber allergy. They do hypo-allergenic household products which include washing-up liquid, fabric softener, soap powder, pre-soak powder, woollens wash and baby soap powder. They also sell a wide variety of unperfumed and dermatologically tested toiletries and a whole range of colour cosmetics.

Ecover products, which can be bought at health food shops and some supermarkets, include toilet cleaner, disinfectant, bleach, cream cleaner for walls and tiles, floor soap, washing powder and heavy-duty hand cleaners.

If you are affected by paint, as so many people are, I recommend International Nursery Paint from Payless.

Remember that a sensitivity to gas or oil is very common, but that you can prove this by having a spell in the summer with everything turned off to see whether you improve. Highly sensitive people may need to move away from their homes to prove this.

Reactions to chemicals are not so difficult to diagnose as they *usually* appear promptly after exposure.

IMMUNITY

See chapter 3 for the best way in which to build up your immune system.

ENCYCLOPEDIA

ABDOMINAL PAIN (ALSO KNOWN AS ABDOMINAL MIGRAINE WHEN ALLERGIC IN ORIGIN)

People may suffer from recurrent abdominal pain with or without other symptoms present. This condition should be thoroughly investigated in order to rule out the possibility of bacteria, intestinal parasites, or even drugs being the cause. Appendicitis must be considered also. In women, abdominal pain may be of gynaecological origin.

If, on investigation, no organic cause can be found, then the cause is likely to be an allergy or intolerance. This, in turn, can result from many different triggers, including gastroenteritis or a long course of antibiotics (both of which remove the good bacteria from the gut) and following a hysterectomy – one reason why more women than men suffer this way. Enzyme deficiencies may also be involved.

Abdominal pain is the number one symptom of gastro-intestinal allergy and is too often dismissed as being emotional in origin (although it is true to say that any form of stress may aggravate an existing allergy). As with most non-specific blood tests used for allergy-induced symptoms, these are always normal, – which is why so many doctors suspect a psychological cause. They seldom think in terms of allergy.

The pain may be localised or general. Usually, but not always, the digestive system as a whole is involved and other symptoms are present. These may include diarrhoea (or constipation), vomiting, nausea, distension (bloating), cramp, wind, blood in stools, etc. When such symptoms are present the condition may be referred to as spastic colon, irritable colon or irritable bowel syndrome.

The most common causes for this allergy are likely to be tap water, milk and milk products, and wheat. Also implicated are white flour, eggs, cheese, chocolate, fish, shellfish, citrus fruits, tomatoes, peanuts, yeast, spices, coffee, apples, bananas, potatoes. Additives known to produce these symptoms include potassium nitrate (E252) and potassium bromate (924) or possibly the gallates (E310–E312). Inhalant allergens which may be responsible include all chemicals, petrol, gas and paint etc.

Abdominal pain in babies (referred to as colic), often considered an unavoidable hazard for the first three months of their lives, is usually a quite unnecessary form of stress for both mother and baby. It is very often caused by the cow's milk formula and may be accompanied by vomiting and/or diarrhoea. Changing to a soya-based formula will often solve the problem. Breast-fed babies who are sufficiently sensitive will also suffer from colic as the milk protein passes from mother to infant. Temporary

A

abstinence from milk and milk products on the part of the mother will put this right. If not diagnosed, this allergy can be aggravated by further allergens when solid foods are introduced.

There is another cause for abdominal pain, and that is coeliac disease. This is caused by a sensitivity to gluten which is present in wheat, oats, barley and rye. The symptoms are loose stools which are foul smelling and tend to float, swollen tummy with accompanied pain and non-thriving in children. On giving up gluten the bowel will return to normal. There is a test to confirm this which involves a biopsy in order to examine the lining of the bowel under a microscope.

Abdominal pain in conjunction with other symptoms can be caused by candidiasis. This is a condition in which a yeast of the natural intestinal flora, known as *Candida albicans*, has multiplied and caused an infection.

See also **Bloating, Candidiasis, Coeliac Disease, Colic** and **Irritable Bowel Syndrome.**

ACHES AND PAINS

The most common cause of muscle pain or stiffness is the result of over-using one's muscles – as in sport or in some exercise or activity not commonly undertaken.

Rheumatism (a general term for any pain affecting the muscles or joints) can be the result of over-exercising or some form of occupational hazard. Nurses are a high-risk group particularly prone to back pain due to the nature of their work.

Tension can cause muscle pain especially in the neck, shoulders and face. Spinal trouble can be another cause. Injuries can lead to rheumatic disorders. Infections such as 'flu and German measles can leave arthritic pains in their wake. These will clear up in due course.

Those people who suffer from aches and pains in any part of their body which do not fit into the above categories may well be suffering from allergy-induced symptoms. Each of the following has a good chance of responding to the dietary approach, otherwise chemical allergens could be involved.

Rheumatoid Arthritis – swollen joints causing pain and stiffness.

Arthralgia – aching joints without apparent inflammation.

Myalgia (also known as Fibrositis) – aching muscles.

The most likely foods to be implicated in these conditions are wheat, milk, citrus fruits, white flour, coffee, tea, chocolate, cola, sugar, beef, pork, cheese, tomatoes, peanuts, food additives (especially colourings) and MSG (monosodium glutamate). Possible inhalant allergens include petrol, gas and paint etc.

See also **Arthritis.**

ACNE

Acne is a hormone-related condition suffered more frequently by people who have an oily skin. It often occurs around puberty and can continue for any length of time, but it usually clears of its own accord in the twenties – even if no cause has been found. It may be aggravated by vitamin deficiencies. For women it can be worse prior to menstruation.

Much can be done to alleviate acne. Sunshine is often found to be beneficial. It helps if you avoid wearing your hair in a fringe. Be wary of lotions, ointments and cosmetics – all of which can cause allergic reactions of the skin and may make your acne worse. Lanolin is a common ingredient used in these preparations to which some people are sensitive. Try to choose non-greasy cosmetics. I would recommend all acne sufferers to use a non-perfumed soap, such as Simple Soap or Boots' Pure Soap. This may be all that is necessary to clear your acne; otherwise you will need to use a medicated soap. Prolonged use of antibiotics should not be used for acne where alternative measures are available. There is much you can do to help yourself.

Foods can often be the cause of acne, and the ones most likely to be involved are milk, sugar, eggs, white flour, coffee, yeast, citrus fruits, cheese, chocolate, artificial colourings, preservatives and other additives. Inhalants, bactericidal agents and drugs have also been implicated. Acne sufferers are sometimes found to be deficient in zinc so a zinc supplement may be helpful.

See also **Dermatitis**.

ADDICTION

The first thing to consider when it becomes obvious that someone is suffering from an addiction is whether this is of psychological origin. Is something wrong in their life? Is the alcohol/drug/nicotine/caffeine/food being used to compensate for some form of stressful life style or maybe just plain boredom? If this is recognised to be so, and some changes can be made for the better, then it should be possible to break the habit.

More often than not this craving is due to an allergy – a masked allergy. This means feeling an immediate boost after taking your drink, cigarette or food. A feeling of well-being pervades the addict (as with a drug) and the knowledge that he/she can now cope with whatever life may bring. Unfortunately this lift will last only a matter of hours, varying with the individual, and depending on the degree of addiction. After this the distressing symptoms will return in whatever form they usually take. They will be accompanied by a low feeling again and a strong urge to return to the 'fix', soon after which they will feel better. This is why it is known as masked allergy. It is the elation/depression syndrome.

With foods such as wheat and corn this will almost always go unre-

A

cognised. In other things it is more obvious. In the case of tobacco it is a reaction to the nicotine. With regard to coffee, tea and cola drinks, it is a reaction to the caffeine. Both are stimulants and, as such, increase alertness and reduce hunger. They can cause insomnia, loss of appetite and weight loss. People can become addicted to a wide range of foods and also to chemicals. In addition, they may suffer from hypoglycaemia (low blood sugar) and feel weak, sweaty, nauseous, shivery, irritable, faint or just plain frustrated before getting their fix.

Addiction is habit forming and, more often than not, has come about without the individual realising it. A lot of willpower is needed in order to break the habit. It should also be recognised that withdrawal symptoms are probably inevitable and can be very unpleasant but, in most cases where allergy is concerned, will be over within a week. Often the third day is the worst, after which the situation improves – although the actual craving takes a good deal longer to dissipate.

The only way to break the habit is not to allow yourself to even think of whatever it is you are addicted to. Keep busy and concentrate entirely on what you are doing. There is a great sense of achievement when you do kick the habit, however, which you well deserve – having proved that you have a strong will. One way of cutting down on the severity of the withdrawal symptoms is to cut the offending item out gradually. Personally, I think that this just prolongs the agony, but it is another option. Don't worry if you return to it in a weak moment. It took me years to give up smoking but I achieved it in the end!

With regard to food allergy addicts, some people eat or drink enormous quantities of their addictant, such as twenty cups of coffee a day. Doctors working in this field believe that over five cups of coffee, or tea, a day denotes allergy. Some people will become more addicted if they have already been exposed to another allergen. You can tell whether you are addicted to something by noting whether you are *really concerned* about running out of it. There is a stronger addictive factor with tobacco than with alcohol (ie, nearly all smokers are addicted; only a few drinkers are).

Among the things to which people can become addicted are drugs (street or medical), nicotine, alcohol, solvents, foods, odours, fumes and chemicals of all kinds. One example of people becoming allergic/addicted to their drugs is when migraine sufferers develop a sensitivity to the commonly prescribed drug, ergotamine. When this happens their migraine will worsen.

Common addictive foods are alcohol, wheat, corn, coffee, tea, cola, milk, chocolate and sugar. (A craving for sweet things is not unusual. We eat far more sugar now that we have ever done in the past.)

See also **Alcohol Dependency** and **Bulimia**.

AGGRESSION

Apart from the obvious reasons for aggression, ie, when the individual is behaving in this manner because he/she feels the circumstances warrant it, there are other involuntary reasons why people exhibit this behaviour. It may be the result of consuming too much alcohol, extreme fatigue, low blood sugar or simply someone's personality due to inherited genes. On the other hand it may be due to allergy.

Dr Albert Rowe, a physician in California, drew attention to work done involving psychosomatic illness in the 1920s. He proved how symptoms such as aggression could be due to a chemical imbalance caused by allergy to foods and chemicals. Dr Richard Mackarness, who worked as a psychiatrist at Park Prewett Hospital in Basingstoke, started getting successes along these lines in the 1970s.

One of the most commonly implicated foods is sugar – cane sugar, not sugar beet. The western world is consuming far more than it did two (or even one) generations ago. Although I can find no reference to it, I remember hearing of a study some years ago carried out on violent prison offenders. They were divided into two groups; one group was put on a sugar-free diet whilst the other continued to eat normally. A substantial number of those on the sugar-free diet calmed down and became less aggressive. When the diets were reversed, the second group calmed down and the first group reverted to their usual aggressive behaviour. Other studies have been done in the USA, one I remember on children, giving similar results.

From the point of view of the allergy sufferer, it seems as if adrenalin starts pumping through the veins and the stomach muscles tighten. The individual feels anything ranging from irritable to violent depending on the degree of the reaction. It is one of the most unfortunate and potentially dangerous – and least understood – forms of allergic reaction.

Apart from sugar, other foods such as milk, wheat, chocolate or food additives may be responsible. Also, a wide range of chemical inhalants – including natural gas, perfumes and even tobacco smoke – can cause this symptom. Trace mineral deficiencies or toxic poisoning can also have this effect.

See also **Violence**.

AGORAPHOBIA

Agoraphobia literally means a fear of open spaces but it is also used to indicate a fear of going outside one's home and, in fact, is normally used in this context. It is a situation which causes the sufferer much anxiety, and in severe cases may result in someone becoming house-bound. Often, this condition is treated with tranquillisers but this is not the long-term answer. It is necessary to discover *why* someone is suffering from agoraphobia.

Anyone who has experienced something very frightening in their past, especially if this occurred outdoors may, quite understandably, develop this type of phobia. Such people can usually be helped by treatment from a psychologist or behavioural therapist.

Allergic people can also suffer total changes in their personalities if the allergic reaction affects their brain. Hence a confident, outgoing person may become nervous, anxious, frightened, weepy, unable to communicate, very stressed and so on. It can require a great act of will, for example, to visit the local shop – this causing much mental effort (or perhaps even proving impossible). This situation is difficult to understand for anyone who has not experienced it. One simply asks that it can be accepted as fact.

Common causes are: coffee, tea, milk, wheat, corn, chemical additives (azo and coal tar dyes in particular), as well as other foods and a whole host of inhaled chemicals.

See also **Claustrophobia**.

ALCOHOL DEPENDENCY

People who feel that they are dependent upon alcohol and would like either to give it up or just have a drink occasionally, need to ask themselves the following questions.

First, are you drinking because you are depressed, lonely or bored? If so, try to change the situation. People can feel very isolated and think that no one cares for them. In fact, people are cared about much more than they ever realise: neighbours, workmates, travelling companions, shopkeepers – all the people with whom you come into contact in your daily life – care about you. Perhaps you can get together from time to time. There are more lonely people than you think. Make the effort to join a club or adult education class or enquire about doing some voluntary work and *get among people.* For housewives bound by children there are toddler groups and the National Housewives Register who would be delighted to have you join them. Many other people feel just as lacking in confidence as you, and once you realise this you will feel much more confident and not need to turn to the bottle any longer.

Secondly, are you drinking because your business/social life seems to require it? If so, then turn to non-alcoholic drinks – offer your own guests one of the wide range of non-alcoholic drinks available for example. More people are drinking less alcohol, and if you feel obliged to give an explanation then 'I'm driving' is acceptable to everyone.

Thirdly, do you keep on drinking because you really crave the stuff? Be honest. It is going to be a hard one to face but, believe me, this business of doing it in secret is a secret to no one. You *can* give it up. You have the guts. You just have to face the fact that you are addicted to it. This may not be as bad as it seems. You are not alone.

Addiction and allergy go hand in hand. That is, addicted people are allergic, but allergic people are not necessarily hooked on their allergen. You may be allergic to alcohol per se, it is true, but you may be allergic to only one of the ingredients. Most alcoholic drinks contain yeast and sugar, and many (but not all) contain artificial additives. Wines and sherries are commonly made from grapes. Red wine also contains an amino acid called tyramine. Cheaper wines contain preservatives and other permitted chemical additives. German wines are usually pretty pure. Beer is always made from hops but also contains other ingredients. 'Lager louts' are undoubtedly drinking too much, but in some cases they are also reacting to an individual ingredient or to one of the many chemical additives. Gin is made from juniper; whisky from wheat, barley or rye; rum from cane sugar. (An addicted whisky drinker may well be in fact a wheat addict rather than an alcohol addict.)

If you feel that you are addicted to alcohol, or to one of the constituents in your favourite tipple, and would like to do something about it, then look under 'Addiction' and consider tackling the problem yourself. Otherwise, you can contact Alcoholics Anonymous who will, I am sure, be very supportive. Better still, do both!

You will find the telephone number of AA in your local directory; otherwise, their general office number is 0904 644026 – where they are open from 9.0am to 5.0pm.

See also **Addiction**.

AMNESIA

Amnesia is a partial or total loss of memory. It is very frightening for the sufferer. It can indicate concussion if memory loss follows an injury to the head. Some serious illnesses can cause amnesia, so a medical check is essential. It can also be caused by an emotional shock (such as a bereavement, for example) which is too distressing for someone to cope with.

Amnesia is also a form of cerebral allergy. The brain (being part of the body) is not exempt from allergic reactions, and this symptom can occur in varying degrees in anyone susceptible to allergic reactions.

If you should find yourself in this predicament, I suggest that you remain quietly in your home and try not to be too distressed. Ask those with whom you live to bear with you and remember, above all, that this condition is *temporary*. It is very frightening but stay quiet and wait and try not to panic. It *will* pass. I advise taking a teaspoonful of sodium bicarbonate in a glass of warm water morning and evening. This will help to disperse your allergic reaction more quickly. Your memory will return all the sooner if you can manage to stay calm.

This symptom may be a delayed reaction from a food or a chemical in a food. Anything up to twenty-four hours following ingestion would not be unusual. If you are reacting to a chemical, such as gas for example, the response is more likely to be a rapid one.

ANAPHYLACTIC SHOCK (ANAPHYLAXIS)

This is a very serious form of allergic reaction but fortunately a rare one. When an antigen (the substance to which someone is sensitive) finds its way into the blood stream (the fastest way being by injection) it will quickly reach the many mast cells all round the body and this will result in releasing large amounts of histamine. Symptoms, which include swelling, appear quickly, and rapid medical attention is required. The situation is most often associated with bee and wasp stings.

Anaphylactic shock means being in a state of shock or collapse. As well as swelling, and a rapid drop in blood pressure, the symptoms include hives, itching, faintness, sweating, nausea and vomiting, weakness, anxiety, confusion, asthma and possibly difficulty in breathing.

Causes include wasp and bee stings and injections of drugs such as penicillin. If you have *ever* reacted in *any* way to penicillin or penicillin-related drugs, you must always mention this to your doctor prior to accepting a prescription.

Further possible causes are artificial additives, especially artificial colourings such as coal-tar dyes, aspirin (aspirin is also a coal-tar derivative), nuts, peanuts (which are not nuts but legumes), cow's milk, eggs, fish and shellfish. Egg-sensitive people should query vaccines. Most vaccines are not now cultivated in egg – beef broth is more commonly used; however, it is safer to check.

People who are very hypersensitive can suffer from anaphylactic shock as a result of medical desensitisation, but this is thought to be very rare. However, if you have ever suffered from any violent allergic reaction, you must always inform your doctor before accepting any form of desensitising injection or, indeed, any injection at all. The same goes for drugs and/or anaesthetics. With regard to anaesthetics, I think it is important to insist upon speaking personally to the anaesthetist before permitting an operation to take place.

There is a school of thought which believes that it is possible that cot-deaths are due to anaphylactic shock when babies encounter cow's milk or eggs etc for the first time.

Anaphylactic shock can appear almost immediately after coming into contact with the antigen or it can be delayed by several hours. Either way, medical attention must be sought rapidly for this life-threatening condition. The standard treatment is a shot of adrenalin and oxygen if required.

See also Cot Deaths.

ANGINA AND ANGINA-TYPE PAIN

Anginal pain is a heavy pain across the upper part of the chest. It can be very severe and may spread down the left arm, up to the chin and even down the right arm. It can be quite overbearing but will probably ease after several minutes. There are various causes of chest pain, some serious. However, angina is caused by atheroma of the coronary arteries. This condition warrants a thorough medical examination. It is brought on by physical activity, walking uphill, cold weather, emotional upsets and smoking, all of which should be avoided if they have been found to cause an attack. Emotional trauma can be responsible for very severe pain. Saturated fats (ie animal fats) and smoking may cause or aggravate an existing condition. The best thing to do is to rest as soon as you feel an attack coming on. In fact it is important to do so.

There are, however, recorded cases of people suffering from the same symptoms with attacks triggered under the same conditions who, when medically examined, have shown no sign of heart disease. When certain foods have been removed from their diets, these attacks have ceased. This has enabled them to return to exercising, venturing out in the cold, etc without experiencing any chest pain. Yet if they were to partake of these same foods again, their pain would return. Foods implicated are wheat, coffee, cow's milk, eggs, fish, shellfish, and artificial colourings such as tartrazine and 154 Brown FK. Other food additives may also be responsible.

See also **Heart Conditions** and **Chest Pains**.

ANGIOEDEMA

This is a condition meaning giant hives associated with swelling which is filled with a watery fluid. When the hives are accompanied by swelling of the mouth and/or other parts of the body, this is known as angioedema. The tongue, throat, lips and, indeed, the whole face may become swollen and the features distorted. This condition is most commonly caused by allergy but can be symptomatic of other serious disorders and should be properly investigated. When the symptoms are of allergic origin, and are severe, medical attention should be sought forthwith as an injection of adrenalin may be required.

Possible allergic causes are widespread – a bee sting or a bite from other insects, penicillin, aspirin or other drugs, foods, food additives such as tartrazine (E102) and other dyes including E110, E122 and E160(b), the benzoate preservatives, sulphur dioxide and a variety of chemical inhalants. Foods which have been implicated include milk and milk products, eggs, nuts, peanuts, fish, shellfish, yeast and strawberries.

In people who probably already have some underlying allergies, sunshine or excessive temperatures of heat or cold can be enough to bring on the unpleasant symptoms of angioedema.

See also **Urticaria** (also known as Hives and Nettlerash).

ANOREXIA NERVOSA

This is a little-understood condition whereby the individual refuses food for fear of putting on weight. Numbers of sufferers are said to be on the increase. Only one in fifteen patients is male. The sufferer convinces herself that she is too fat, needs to lose weight and does not need food. She continues in this manner until she is very underweight but believes this not to be so and will not listen to family and friends who try to help. If persuaded to eat against her will, she may secretly cause herself to vomit all the food she has taken. Eventually, hormonal changes will cause her periods to stop and she will suffer from anaemia. Family rows will inevitably develop as a result of all the anxiety she is causing.

This is a very depressing time for the patient's family. It may last from a few months to a number of years. No one really understands the cause but it is thought to be, at least in some cases, a cry for help. Perhaps discussion of her worries, and arrangements for a change in life style when she has recovered may be an encouragement.

Psychiatric help is needed, with the possibility of hospitalisation. In-patient treatment consists of being confined to bed, given drugs to increase the appetite and reduce anxiety, and a weight-gaining diet. Extra nutrients in the form of vitamin and mineral supplements will be valuable to correct the inevitable deficiencies.

No one has suggested a link between aneroxia nervosa and food allergy and, at this stage, I cannot see where a connection could be made, but I do not think the possibility should be ruled out. What I do know, without doubt, is that some genuinely food-allergic people have been wrongly diagnosed as anorexic. When a genetically disposed hypersensitive person has, through no fault of his own, reached a low ebb, physically, mentally or emotionally, he becomes highly susceptible to developing a whole range of sensitivities. To discover that you are becoming intolerant to one food after another is a most frightening experience because, apart from the self-discipline required not to eat, every normal person knows that you have to eat in order to stay alive.

In fact much can be done to help people in this predicament by introducing them to seldom-consumed foods which they are more likely to be able to tolerate, advising them to rotate these so as not to become sensitised to them, and at the same time showing them how to build up their immune system in order to regain a tolerance to those foods they have lost.

However, few people are likely to obtain this information from their GP – who may well not have come across a case of multiple food allergy before. He sees a patient who has lost weight and is claiming that she cannot eat anything; she will undoubtedly be worried and anxious, so quite understandably, the doctor thinks in terms of anorexia. This in turn will cause the patient much distress, knowing that whoever goes along with this diagnosis will want her to eat the very foods she knows to be the cause of her illness. This sort of situation would seem to justify the expense of visiting a doctor working in the field of allergy and environmental illness.

See also **Multiple Food Allergies** and **Myalgic Encephalomyelitis (ME)**.

ANXIETY

Anxiety can cause people to feel depressed, weak, listless, tense, nervous,

A

irritable, tearful and give them sleepless or broken nights. It may also be accompanied by headaches, pains in any part of the body, nausea, diarrhoea, palpitations and so on. Symptoms of anxiety should be reported to the doctor if only to eliminate any possibility of serious disease.

Life is a real challenge – for all of us some of the time and for some of us all of the time, or so it may seem. We worry about everything from relationships to jobs to children and a million other things. Just keeping our heads above water, physically, emotionally and financially can be quite a strain. For the majority of us these anxieties will come in phases and then the situation will ease – until the next crisis!

Those people for whom there seems no respite, unless they are very strong, may suffer chronic symptoms of anxiety (commonly described as 'stress') and eventually something has to give. The obvious answer is to change the circumstances which have caused the stress but this, so often, is simply not practicable. Luckily we have services and associations to whom people can turn to get a break when everything becomes too much. For those people already at a low ebb, the smallest worry, normally taken in their stride, can cause acute anxiety.

Doctors may prescribe a tranquilliser or sedative, and for a short-term solution, when things seem quite desperate, you may be grateful to take up this offer. However, tranquillisers should never be considered anything but a temporary measure to get you back on your feet. Don't drink if you are on tranquillisers, and check before taking any other drugs.

However, what about anxiety when you have nothing in your life to be anxious about? You are not over-worked. You have no family or financial worries. You keep looking for an explanation for your anxiety but nothing emerges.

For women, the reason, if it is intermittent, may be due to pre-menstrual syndrome (PMS) or it may be caused by taking the Pill, which alters the hormone balance. Anxiety in either sex may even be caused by not eating a properly balanced diet – thus causing a lack of nutrients. Alternatively, it can be due to a deficiency of trace minerals – namely zinc, magnesium or calcium – or a lack of vitamins, particularly B complex vitamins, vitamin C and vitamin E.

Anxiety may also be allergy-induced – in fact it very often is. It can accompany other illnesses, migraine for instance which, in turn, is a sensitivity to something. It is commonly related to a caffeine sensitivity.

Foods most often incriminated include coffee, tea, cola, chocolate, milk, wheat, other grains, eggs, sugar, cheese, citrus fruits and artificial additives, particularly the azo dyes such as tartrazine (E102) and amaranth (E123). A whole range of inhalants may be responsible – perfumes, gas, fumes from oil, coal, tobacco, car fumes, cleaning materials and other chemicals used in home, garden, job or hobby.

See also **Brain Allergies, the Pill** and **Pre-menstrual Syndrome (PMS)**.

A

ARTHRITIS

Arthritis is a general term for inflammation of the joints. Acute arthritis is rare and may follow injury or bacterial infection. The two main forms of chronic arthritis are rheumatoid arthritis and osteo-arthritis. They are both progressive diseases of the joints affecting mainly the hips, knees, spine or finger joints.

Rheumatoid arthritis consists of swollen, painful joints – warm to the touch – and stiffness which is usually at its worst in the morning. It used to be considered unlikely to start until young middle age or middle age but now it is not uncommon for children to suffer from it. Anaemia can develop as a result. Blood tests may confirm the condition.

Osteo-arthritis is a disorder affecting more women than men and is considered to be due to the wear and tear of ageing. It can begin during the menopause. If the joints are damaged by injury, arthritis can set in. If can also be a by-product of another illness, such as German measles, but if this is the case it will clear up of its own accord.

With both forms of arthritis it is believed that the risk is increased by overweight. It has been steadily increasing since the beginning of the century, and now seven to eight million people suffer from arthritis in this country. The typical British diet is undoubtedly an underlying cause.

Special exercises will help this condition. Physiotherapists can advise here. Blood tests and X-rays should be carried out to eliminate other disorders. A diet high in fish and/or the taking of cod-liver oil or halibut-liver oil capsules is said to help. B complex vitamins are helpful, too, as is 1g of vitamin C daily. The latter is especially helpful for people who take aspirin, as aspirin counteracts the vitamin C in your diet.

There are many arthritis drugs around, most of which will produce side-effects – especially if taken on a long-term basis. Opren, a drug widely used at one time, had to be withdrawn from use when it was found to be doing damage in other directions. It is usually found that drugs only partially suppress arthritic symptoms. Steroids should be used only for advanced cases when there is no alternative, because of adverse effects. Joint replacements can be made on affected joints, the most commonly done being hip replacements, with a high success rate.

The great majority of those arthritis sufferers who have been on properly monitored elimination diets have often been able to prove a food (or foods) to be responsible for their symptoms. Scientific double-blind trials have been conducted world-wide, and have proved this, but the British medical profession is notoriously stubborn in accepting anything 'new'.

Arthritis is sometimes accompanied by other complaints which may be of allergic origin but which have been treated as separate symptoms. Orthodox medicine believes that arthritis may 'come and go' with periods of remission. It also believes that arthritis sufferers are susceptible to placebo effects. This is inconsistent. How can you tell whether a placebo effect is just that and not the 'going' of a 'coming and going' period?

If fact, food allergy can be proved to be the cause of arthritis over and over again with elimination diets and challenge tests.

The most commonly incriminated food is cow's milk and its products, after which come wheat, corn, cheese, coffee, tea, yeast, chocolate, citrus fruits, sugar, pork, food additives, especially colourings, monosodium glutamate and sodium nitrite.

I have not been able to find any research which implicates chemical allergy, but this does not rule out the possibility – especially in cases where people are working with chemicals.

See also **Aches and Pains**.

ASTHMA

A severe attack of asthma is frightening to behold. It is even more frightening to experience. You feel as if you are suffocating, and the panic induced by this aggravates the attack. It will help if the bystander can assure the sufferer that he will make contact with the person closest to the patient. In the case of a child, this is likely to be the mother. However for an adult, too, it will be enormously reassuring if whoever they have most confidence in can be with them. Probably only someone who has actually experienced a severe attack themselves will realise the *vital* importance of this. Before this can be accomplished, emergency steps have to be taken. Reassure the patient, yourself, that he will be alright, and take all practical steps to ensure that he is. Keep calm, as any anxiety on your part will relay itself to the sufferer. He should be sitting upright. Put pillows behind him if necessary and make sure he uses his inhaler and/or whatever medication he has been prescribed for just such an emergency. Help him to administer this because he should not exert any energy himself. Make sure that he has fresh air – open the nearby windows.

Patients developing a bad attack may need early and urgent hospital admission. In a severe attack the patient becomes mentally confused, is unable to talk, exhibits a blue tinge on lips and tongue, and has a pulse rate rise to about 120. If in any doubt, dial for an ambulance or drive the patient quickly to a hospital emergency department. However, there is a wide range of treatments available which could help avoid this extreme situation arising.

In severe cases doctors may recommend the use of a nebuliser. This is a very effective and rapid way of relieving the symptoms of asthma.

A less severe but nevertheless disabling attack will consist of a cough – more prevalent at night – difficult breathing, wheezing, a fast pulse and the possibility of vomiting. A milder form of asthma will be a persistent cough and breathlessness with little or no wheezing.

Attacks can occur suddenly following exposure to an allergen, or they

A

may develop slowly – manifesting themselves some hours later. The latter form can prove equally severe.

Asthma can start at any age – childhood, adolescence or later. It is not uncommon for children to develop it around the age of three. Most of them will outgrow this in their teens although, being susceptible, they will always have to be on the look-out for other allergies developing. Ten per cent of children are said now to be born asthmatic. It affects more boys than girls. In March, 1990, the *Daily Telegraph* quoted a report saying that the number of people suffering from asthma is rising and could be as many as two million. The report said that, for adults aged fifteen to sixty-four, 'preventable factors' contributed to death in four out of five cases. The report, issued by the Office of Health Economics, said 'There is evidence that preventive treatment remained under-prescribed.'

Try to balance your child's life style. Let him work within his own limits. He is the best guide as to what and how much he can achieve. Never think your child is 'putting on' an asthma attack. It is not worth the risk. Fatalities can occur but numbers are extremely low. Hormonal changes, such as pregnancy or menstruation, can provoke an attack when there is already an underlying cause; endocrine imbalance can also provoke an attack.

The biggest myth about asthma is the belief that emotions can be the cause of attacks. Luckily, most people, including doctors, are becoming better informed and realising that this is not so. Asthma attacks always have a physical, not an emotional, cause (or combination of causes). However, in someone already suffering from an underlying allergy, any stress trigger, emotional or otherwise, can be enough to tip the balance. The converse applies also, in that when someone is already under stress, a smaller amount than usual of the particular allergen is all that is necessary to start an attack. This applies to other allergies as well, but especially to asthma. Emotional upsets make things worse but are seldom the only cause. A happy family life and relief of stress will help the sufferer a great deal because emotional factors lower general resistance and can cause respiratory changes which can more readily lead to an asthma attack when an allergen presents itself.

Although asthma is mainly an allergic disease, viral or bacterial in-fections can cause inflammation (and therefore narrowing) of the tubes and will induce asthma in susceptible people. Children are more prone to viruses as they have not yet had a chance to build up their immunity. Colds can lead to coughing and wheezing. The membranes lining the tubes and air spaces of the lungs become increasingly irritated; this provides an ideal environment for bacteria or the germs which cause bronchitis. If the patient develops a chest infection, this too will worsen the asthma. It follows, therefore, that asthma attacks can follow other infections also. In some people asthma may be associated *only* with respiratory infections. Such people suffer from asthma which is caused by infections rather than allergy. They should seek prompt medical attention for coughs and colds.

Similarly, in others, asthma symptoms may be brought on only by exercise, cold weather, dampness and so on. Their over-sensitive airways react to these stimuli by narrowing. Once they stop exercising or remove themselves from the damaging environment, their asthma will abate in a relatively short time. Any of these situations can aggravate an underlying allergy to other things. So often these present themselves in combination.

The most common form of asthma, therefore, is allergy-induced asthma. The term 'extrinsic asthma' means entering the body from outside. The term 'intrinsic' means inside the body (hereditary disposition, state of immune system, etc); this term is now used less often as doctors realise that there always has to be an external trigger, too – something the patient has eaten, drunk, inhaled or been injected with. People who wheeze constantly are allergic to something they are coming into contact with all the time ie house dust. Although this condition is sometimes treated with steroids it is better to try to improve the environment, discover the cause or causes through reliable testing and try to be desensitised.

Always have your inhaler and/or other prescribed medical treatments to hand wherever you go. If you come into contact with something you know will trigger an attack, such as cigarette smoke, say so, and avoid it at all costs. If this is quite impossible, do make use of modern drugs. If in doubt, consult your doctor.

The inhaled types of drugs are considered quick, safe and the most effective. They are less likely to contain colouring agents and other causes of side-effects. For severe reactions, cortisone – a steroid – works quickly and there are few side-effects when used on a one-off basis; in long-term use it will cause irreversible side-effects such as moon-face, excess hair and so on. Nevertheless, cortisone is very effective, and its use must be balanced against the patient's needs. *Intal* (sodium cromoglycate) is an excellent preventative, safe and free from side-effects as it is not absorbed into the blood stream. It can be tolerated by most people. When asthma is anticipated (such as when visiting a house where there is a cat, for example) a cat-sensitive person can take a puff of *Intal* and go visiting without fear of developing asthma – in most cases. *Intal* stabilises the mast cells, which are one of the many types of cells making up the immune system. Antihistamines are generally regarded as being not so effective except for pollen-induced asthma. Orthodox tests are reasonably accurate for the limited number of allergens available, but are no good for foods. Orthodox desensitisation is disappointing for asthmatics, but the intradermal testing and neutralisation used by many clinical ecologists is good – as is EPD (enzyme-potentiated desensitisation) used by others. Sleeping tablets should not be taken by asthmatics. Caution should be used with all drugs, and those with artificial colourings should be avoided. Aspirin is a common offender and can cause serious asthma attacks. It is safer to use paracetamol if a pain killer is needed.

A

Peak-flow meters can be prescribed or bought. These provide a means of gauging the degree of breathlessness in a patient, and therefore indicate whether or not medical treatment is required. For safety's sake, always carry your inhaler with you.

We have discussed asthma caused by infections and sensitivities to temperature changes and climatic conditions. Now we come to the most common cause of asthma – allergens. In this illness inhalant allergens are even more common than food allegens. Any of the following or any combination of the following may be responsible for an asthma attack. Any sort of dust or pollen should be avoided by asthmatics, whether or not they are a cause, because they are likely to aggravate the condition. Pollen sensitivity is very common, and even a few grains can spark off a severe attack. Grass, flowers and trees all produce pollen. Seasonal asthma between February and May is likely to be caused by tree pollens; asthma from early June to mid-July will be caused by grass pollen, and asthma from July to November may well be caused by mould spores. Watch out for pine trees at Christmas. Many allergic people are affected by pine.

The one thing all allergists agree upon is the detrimental effect of cigarette smoke upon the asthmatic. Not only should he not smoke himself but other people's cigarette smoke should be avoided at all costs. Luckily for asthmatics smoking has become socially unacceptable in most places so it is now easier to avoid.

Other possible causes of asthma include woollen clothes and blankets, feather pillows, duvets and cushions, house-dust mites in carpets and bedding, and horse-hair mattresses and sofas. Watch out also for dogs, cats, birds, rabbits, horses and hamsters. (The only pets you can really be sure of being safe with are fish.) Don't be in a hurry to get rid of your pet, though. The cause of the asthma may not even be the pet itself – it could be his bedding or even his food, and these can be changed. Great distress can be caused to the asthma sufferer – as well as to the pet – if you get rid of the pet, so do find out first whether there is another answer, such as being desensitised to the allergen, before you do anything drastic. You may even be mistaken, and there could be another cause altogether.

Other causes of asthma include household fumes such as gas, oil, coal, wood fires,etc, industrial fumes, traffic fumes, paint, creosote, wood preservatives, air fresheners, aerosol sprays, cavity wall insulation, synthetic fabrics, solvents, varnishes, soft plastics, household cleaners, detergents, disinfectants, washing up liquid, perfumes, perfumed soaps, cosmetics, toiletries (men's as well as women's), indoor plants, chemicals used in the garden or in nursery gardens, farm chemicals (including aerial sprays), moulds (found in old houses) and environmental pollution of any kind. There are many occupational hazards, and the asthmatic should definitely not go for a job which would bring him into contact with grains or straw or sawdust or any other form of dust particles. Likewise, he should avoid working in places such as hairdressers, dry cleaners or anywhere where chemicals of any kind are in constant use.

A final but important point is that it is essential that an asthmatic (or his parent) talks to the anaesthetist before undergoing an operation and that his history of asthma is thoroughly discussed.

Foods and drinks can be (and very often are) implicated in an asthma attack either singly, together, or in combination with one or more inhalants. The most common one, certainly in infants and possibly in everyone else, is cow's milk. Most baby formulas are made from cow's milk, a product which was intended by Nature for calves and is therefore not always suitable for human infants. Other suspect foods include eggs, cheese, wheat, corn, yeast, fish, pork, peanuts, nuts, spices, citrus fruits, chocolate, peas, beans, beef, onion and tomatoes. Some people's sensitivity is such that even the odours to these foods can trigger an asthma attack.

Alcoholic and non-alcoholic drinks are made from many different products, and they include preservatives and other chemical additives, all of which are possible causes of asthma. Salt, MSG (monosodium glutamate), artificial colourings (particularly tartrazine and other azo dyes), preservatives (especially the benzoates), sulphur dioxide (many asthmatics are sulphur-sensitive), traces of antibiotics found in meat, eggs and milk are all additional potential hazards for the asthma sufferer.

Beware of the following additives. And there are others which have not been so well researched but which, without doubt, affect the individual, E102, 107, E110, E122, E123, E124, E131, E142, 155, E210, E211, E212, E213, E214, E215, E216, E217, E218, E219, E220, E221, E222, E223, E224, E249, E250, E310, E311, E312. E11, sodium benzoate, and E223, sodium metabisulphite, are used in orange squash.

Be wary of all drugs which, unlike foods, are not marked with a list of their ingredients. Artificial colourings which can trigger asthma, hyperactivity and many other allergies are still widely used in drugs – including anti-allergy drugs; this shows the ignorance surrounding ingested allergens and the hazards which allergic people face. (Until recent years, Piriton, a widely-used anti-histamine, was coloured with tartrazine!). Luckily, some people are on our side, and Boots the Chemist does a range of colour-free medicines for children. (Adults, perhaps, are expected not to suffer from the problem!)

Penicillin and penicillin-related drugs may cause asthma, but there are alternative antibiotics which can be prescribed. Make sure that you avoid those with artificial colourings. Aspirin and aspirin-containing drugs can cause a serious reaction so, if in any doubt, paracetamol should be used as an alternative.

As an asthmatic you need to take advantage of those modern medical drugs specifically designed for this purpose. There are now some excellent ones available which will help to keep your asthma under control. You also need to be your own physician. By that I mean you must plan your lifestyle and use of drugs to your best advantage. At all times you will need to keep your head, not be afraid to speak out if necessary, and maybe make rapid decisions in emergencies.

A

Regulate your life, avoiding stress whenever you can. Learn to breathe properly. Many people, especially asthmatics, breathe by heaving their chests up and down instead of pushing their diaphragms gently in and out in the correct manner. If you are conscious that you do not breathe properly, then you will greatly benefit by having lessons from a physiotherapist or by going to relaxation classes. Either way you will learn to relax and this is very important. Hypnotherapy has proved good for asthmatics also but do go to a medically trained hypnotherapist who has been personally recommended. Swimming is good for breathing control and the warm air around the pool is ideal for those asthmatically inclined. Should you find that you are affected by the chlorine or other disinfectant, you can take an antihistamine or other allergy drug beforehand. If this does not do the trick, make enquiries regarding another swimming pool in your district and check whether they use a different disinfectant. It is good to take what exercise you can but avoid physically pushing yourself too far – and only *you* are the best judge of this.

To summarise, keep yourself away from all known irritants and always check your foods. Vacuum your bedroom daily and your mattress also (unless you prefer to cover it with plastic). Sunshine and dry air are good for getting rid of dust mites. Remove yourself from all external allergens as far as possible. Try to avoid contact with infection; take a good healthy diet with necessary supplements and get plenty of fresh air and sufficient exercise to suit your needs. Instead of dusting, wipe your furniture with a damp cloth. Avoid brushing if possible and wear a mask when hoovering and in all other dusty situations. This mask is also useful to keep the air warm for people who get asthma through breathing in cold air. These medical masks can be obtained from chemist shops. Alternatively, wearing a scarf over the nose and mouth warms the air first so that the lungs and respiratory passages are less affected. Deep breathing in clean, non-polluted air is good, as are walking, dancing and swimming. Air filters and ionisers will improve the quality of the air in your home. Ionisers can be bought for the car too.

Extra nutrients in the form of supplements help to counteract all the unavoidable toxins. Those recommended are:

Vitamin C, 1g, 1–3 times daily
A strong preparation of B complex vitamins or multi-vitamins
Strong multi-mineral supplement
Evening Primrose Oil 250mg, 1–3 times daily
Vitamin E 500iu daily

This regime will help to boost your immune system and raise your allergy tolerance level, thereby making you less subject to asthma than you otherwise would be.

I suffered from asthma as a child, and I know how cruel and disabling it can be and the terror of a really severe attack. My heart goes out to those who are afflicted this way and I hope very much that you will find that at least some of this information will help to alleviate your symptoms. See also **Bronchitis, Breathlessness.**

AUTISM, ALLERGY-INDUCED

The following is taken from the Allergy-Induced Autism Support and Self-Help Group leaflet, and is reproduced with their kind permission.

We call it allergy-induced autism, and indeed the majority of the children in our Group have allergies to many foods/chemicals, the main ones being wheat, milk and salicylates. But it is more complex than that. I strongly believe these children's metabolism is so hay-wire that a combination of their own body chemicals makes them behave in an autistic manner.

So what are the signs and symptoms? They may be any combination of the following. Not being aware of the world; lack of eye contact; general learning disability; difficulty in relating to other people; hyperactivity; being withdrawn and miserable; repetitive behaviour; fixation on one subject; sleep problems and being anxious or afraid.

Such children are also likely to display odd behaviour of which the following are typical examples: eating strange substances – eg, earth, sand, rubber, paper etc. Spinning things obsessively, spinning themselves, touching smooth objects compulsively, fascination with lights, arms flapping when excited, jumping up and down, walking on tip-toes and giggling or screaming for no apparent reason.

The majority of this group of children develop *perfectly normally* until the age of approximately eighteen months to two years with *no sign of any abnormality.*

Through studying many questionnaires sent out to our parents regarding their children's eating habits, cravings, dislikes etc, and their familial history concerning allergies, drugs given to the children and mothers during pregnancy, I find a consistent pattern which shows that most of the children eat or crave foods/other substances containing phenolic compounds or derivatives of this. The colourings that make them react so badly contain phenols, as do plastics, paper, rubber and seventy per cent of all foods. It is hardly surprising, therefore, that they seem to be allergic to many things!

I am sure that many of the enzymes in these children are malfunctioning due to the effects of phenolic compounds which I believe to be blocking the pathways. This may be confirmed by the fact that children whose amino acid pathways have been tested were found to be low in certain amino acids and high in others – surely this indicates a malfunction somewhere?

Alcohol contains pyrogallol, which is a phenol, and when you think of the damage alcohol can do it is not hard to see how

A

these children can malfunction. Of course, they presumably have a genetic predisposition to this type of problem (hence the allergic family) or every child would become autistic when exposed to these substances. Some also display a tendency towards hypoglycaemia (low blood sugar) and possibly other slight physical malfunctions.

We know from documented research, that these children have altered levels of dopamine and serotonin in their blood. This is understandable if a child does not possess the correct enzyme to convert these substances to their next step or to deactivate them after use. They will then circulate in the body and possibly react with phenolic compounds to form morphine-like and similar substances within the child's own body.

I am so convinced that this is definitely a part of their problem, in which case our children are just 'junkies' of their own body chemicals.

If this is part or all of the cause of their problems, then it would indicate why they start to improve when the offenders are removed from their diets and also why they respond to vitamin/mineral therapy. But they do need exorbitant amounts of vitamins to cope with getting body levels to normal as most of their stores are either blocked by the toxic substances or are being used to detoxify.

I must stress that this is *only a hypothesis* and is based purely upon observing my own child and on information from parents of similar children, together with my own research into the subject. However, it would be nice to be able to have this hypothesis examined to see whether it may be a possibility. If so, then perhaps it may be relatively easy to correct and, therefore, make our children's and our own lives as parents, much more enjoyable.

BACKACHE

Backache is one of the most common ailments. Most people suffer from it at some time in their lives. Overweight and tall people are said to be at greatest risk. However painful, it is not usually a symptom of some more serious disease and, given time, it nearly always clears up of its own accord. This type of back pain is mechanical in origin and is helped by rest. In fact, heat, rest and painkillers are the orthodox forms of treatment. Daily exercises are also recommended, and those people dogged enough to pursue them undoubtedly benefit. Strengthening tummy muscles relieves part of the load which is otherwise passed down to the back.

A slipped disc is a common cause of back pain and may occur after lifting, gardening or similar strain. It is more common after the age of twenty-five. Slipped discs cause pain in the lower part of the back which may spread down the legs. This pain may be severe and will be made worse by bending, standing up suddenly or even coughing. Home treatment is resting on a firm bed (or even the floor in severe cases), pain-killers, and heat applied to the affected area.

However, anyone suffering back pain for more than a day or two without improvement should consult their doctor to eliminate other less common specific disorders; he may advise an X-ray.

Some women always suffer from backache at the beginning of a period; others do from time to time.

Pain in the kidney area (with or without cystitis) can be caused by stones or infection. If infection, this will show up on analysis of a urine specimen. Equally, it can be of allergic origin – particularly if it is associated with other symptoms of allergy. Backache is sometimes present, along with other aches and pains, as part of the withdrawal symptoms of an elimination diet; backache can be an allergic reaction in its own right.

The most likely food allergen is cow's milk but any other foods or food additives can be implicated.

A calcium supplement, either on its own or combined with magnesium in the form of dolomite, can be helpful to chronic back pain sufferers.

BALANCE, LOSS OF

Loss of balance may be caused by a variety of conditions, occasionally serious. If it is more than momentary, or recurs, medical advice should be sought. It is not uncommon in the elderly.

Among the more common causes of this symptom are anaemia, excess alcohol, dizziness and feeling faint. Less commonly considered is a symptom of sensitivity to food, or inhalants. Extremes of temperature or sudden temperature changes may cause a temporary feeling of

B

faintness. Low blood pressure is another possible cause of dizziness and fainting spells, all of which can lead to loss of balance.

See also **Dizziness** and **Fainting Attacks**.

BLISTERS

Blisters are caused either as the result of an injury to the outside of the body, such as a burn, or by friction, such as, for example, the rubbing of the back of an ill-fitting shoe against the heel. Try not to let the blisters burst. If this should happen, however, burst blisters must be kept clean and free from infection. When a blister does become infected, medical treatment should be sought.

Some infectious diseases, such as shingles, will cause blisters, but these should be readily diagnosed due to the form they take and accompanying symptoms.

There are some serious causes of blistering, so if in doubt, consult your doctor.

Some forms of eczema produce blisters and these may be described as contact eczema when they are due to something with which the body is coming into contact. For example, blisters on the hands could be caused by an adverse reaction to detergents, soap powders or toiletries. Allergies to metals are not uncommon. Many people react to nickel, which is the metal used for the cheaper forms of jewellery. Most people will find they are safe with gold, silver or platinum. There are plenty of anti-allergy creams which can be prescribed but usually the cause of contact allergy is not too hard to detect. Rubber allergy is another one which springs to mind, and people thus affected will need to substitute their rubber gloves and wellies for those made of PVC.

Very often eczema in the form of blisters is not a contact allergy but is caused by a reaction to a food, drink or additive.

One form of allergy most commonly mistaken for contact allergy involves the occurrence of a crop of tiny blisters on babies' bottoms. Of course, this can be due to a cream or talcum powder, to something impregnated in a disposable nappy, or to the soap powder used for washing a terry towelling nappy, but it is more than likely to be due to a reaction to a food – such as milk or eggs.

See also **Eczema** and **Mouth Ulcers**.

BLOATING (OF THE STOMACH)

This symptom can have several causes. The most common cause is a natural reaction, experienced by everyone, which is due to specific properties in certain foods, especially beans such as haricot beans used in the preparation of baked beans.

Bloating is also a symptom of coeliac disease; in this case it will be accompanied by other classic symptoms and can be detected by a test.

Candidiasis is another condition which causes bloating, but, again, will be accompanied by other symptoms.

However, bloating following the ingestion of food (not necessarily immediately) is caused by a food intolerance, most commonly to wheat, eggs or milk. The stomach swells in total disproportion to the amount of food which has been consumed. To give an extreme example, it is possible to eat one peanut and go up two dress sizes within a short space of time. This makes someone appear to be in the advanced stages of pregnancy. Not only is this a highly embarrassing symptom (especially, one presumes, for men) but it is also very uncomfortable, much more so than actually being pregnant – when one is permitted to stretch in gradual stages.

When swelling occurs all over the body, and does not dissipate fairly rapidly, it is essential to consult your doctor as this is an entirely different situation and could be due to kidney disease or hypothyroidism. Similarly, this can happen as the result of a severe allergic reaction requiring immediate medical attention.

See also **Abdominal Pain**, **Candidiasis**, and **Coeliac Disease**.

BLOOD PRESSURE, HIGH (HYPERTENSION)

This is a condition which rarely causes symptoms, so for those people over thirty-five years of age it is a good idea to have their blood pressure checked every few years as high blood pressure can lead to serious complications.

Some related causes include obesity, heavy drinking, smoking and the contraceptive pill and, in rare cases, kidney disease. (Even the slightly overweight are more at risk than those of average weight.) When overweight people go on a diet of good, fresh, natural foods they usually find that their blood pressure, as well as weight, becomes lower. Exercise also plays a part.

Whilst there is no doubt that inherited genes play a major role in susceptibility to developing high blood pressure, there is much the individual can do to help himself. Giving up alcohol and smoking is recommended. You are also advised to decrease your sugar and salt intake, eliminate caffeine, avoid stress and take regular exercise.

Foods believed to help reduce blood pressure include egg yolks, green leafy vegetables, yeast, liver, wheat germ, onions and garlic. In other words this means a good healthy diet including plenty of fresh fruit and vegetables and replacing animal fats with vegetable oils. Lots of lightly cooked vegetables cooked in the minimum of water – in order to retain their vitamins – are best. Avoid too many processed foods as these usually contain a good deal of salt. Carbohydrate foods are implicated in high blood pressure, especially those containing refined sugar and starch.

There is much controversy in the medical world regarding the part played by salt in the incidence of high blood pressure. There is no doubt that populations which use more salt have a higher rate and those which

B

consume less have a lower rate. Nevertheless, there is a school of thought which believes that our own individual susceptibility to developing high blood pressure, as a result of a higher intake of salt, varies. I would go along with this because the whole concept of food intolerance proves that we react on an individual basis to everything we eat. Why should salt be an exception?

Which ever way you look at it, it is a fact that in the western world high blood pressure is known to rise with age, so it is well worth taking the measures one can before resorting to drugs. I would suggest that cutting down on salt is preferable to cutting it out of our diets completely (unless you choose to use a salt substitute) as we do need to keep the sodium balance in our bodies. An increase in your potassium intake would be beneficial but this must be checked if you are on drugs. Calcium, B complex vitamins, garlic perles and vitamin E are all recommended, but the vitamin E dosage should be built up gradually, starting from 100iu daily.

When there is no arteriosclerosis or kidney disease, high blood pressure can be assumed to be caused by an allergy (or, if you prefer it, your own individual susceptibility), either to something you are eating, drinking or, if you are a smoker, to smoking – or perhaps to a combination of any of these.

To sum up, the most likely foods, by far, are caffeine-containing products which are tea, coffee, chocolate, cola drinks and some over-the-counter medications for colds, 'flu and headaches etc designed to give you a temporary pep-up in order to cajole you into believing that they are an effective 'cure'. Any food, however, can cause high blood pressure, and having your blood pressure checked before and after going onto an elimination diet should prove this point.

Certain additives are implicated in this condition, in particular Indigo Carmine (E132) and sulphur dioxide (E220).

It is also possible to suffer from low blood pressure, but this is relatively rare. Although it is better to have a low blood pressure than a high one, people whose blood pressure is too low may suffer from dizziness and fainting spells.

Aspirin is one of the best preventive measures for avoiding high blood pressure which can, in turn, lead to a stroke. However, it should only be taken on a daily basis by those people at risk and on the recommendation of your doctor. Garlic perles are said by some medical authorities to reduce high blood pressure by neutralising the toxins in the intestines. Also, it is said that eating grapefruit helps to bring down the blood pressure.

BRAIN ALLERGIES (EFFECTS OF ALLERGY ON THE BRAIN)

We know that people may suffer physical symptoms, such as headaches or diarrhoea, when they are under stress. Such pressures can also lead to mental symptoms such as depression or anxiety, and extreme or prolonged stress can lead to physical or mental breakdown. These external pressures are well understood and documented. In fact it is quite acceptable to tell your doctor the cause in such circumstances. For example, your GP is likely to be sympathetic if you should say 'I am feeling dreadfully depressed, doctor. My father died six months ago and I just cannot come to terms with losing him.'

The fact that we all have different breaking points is due to our differing hereditary dispositions and our own mental and physical resources at any given time. No one ever knows what internal stresses another person has to contend with, thus making it impossible for us to justify judging one another. It may require far more courage for one person to walk down the street than for another to jump off the high diving board.

Allergies also affect everyone differently and in varying degrees. They can affect the skin, the gut, the joints – any part of the body, in fact, including the brain. Why indeed should the brain be exempt? Yet, the ignorance of the medical profession as a whole in this, the twentieth century, is such that, with few exceptions, doctors are quite unable to grasp the fact that the brain can be affected by food. They do not learn about brain allergies in their medical training so, *ipso facto*, they do not exist! If your allergies appear in the form of a rash or wheezing, you may get a correct diagnosis – if you are lucky. However, try telling your doctor that milk causes you to be depressed and, as likely as not, you will be branded as neurotic or paranoid. It is quite acceptable to say that you are *suffering* from depression but, in this instance, it is definitely not in your interests to know the reason why!

The cause and effect of food allergies affecting the brain have been well documented in medical journals since the 1920s. In fact, the subject was documented as far back as the seventeenth century by Robert Burton who regarded certain foods as 'engendering melancholy humours in the body' and wrote that 'all that comes from milk increases melancholy' in his *Anatomy of Melancholy*.

Nowadays such problems are usually labelled as psychosomatic, and patients are offered psychiatric treatment often involving tranquillisers and other drugs. I have come across some horrific stories from people who have been in-patients in mental hospitals and have been so drugged that they became total zombies when they were simply sensitive to a food or inhalant. Those people I have talked to have, at some point in their lives, 'escaped' to tell the tale. How many more, I wonder, have not?

Considering that the Freudian psychoanalytical approach to mental illness has produced such poor results over the years, one would think it would have been discredited by now. What of the scientific explanation of cause and effect which can be so eminently demonstrated in the allergy approach? With the exception of a few doctors who have the guts to stand up for what they believe in, the British Medical Association does not want to know.

I tell you this. If every mental home or home for maladjusted or disturbed children were to put their patients on a diet of fresh meat, fruit and vegetables with only pure water to drink, and provide a controlled environment (see introduction), within two weeks they would see some remarkable results and thereby end a nightmare existence for at least some of their patients and bring hope and joy to their families for years to come.

So what sort of symptoms might you get with brain allergies? The most common are anxiety and depression. However, more severe ones – such as psychosis, paranoia and schizophrenia – have also been attributed, at least in part, to food. The tension/fatigue syndrome is well known; this causes the brain to become overactive with no let up – the patient naturally soon becoming mentally exhausted. Other symptoms which can be caused by allergic reactions and which can affect adults or children are: loss of energy, extreme fatigue, sleepiness, feeling drugged, lack of libido, confusion, amnesia, panic attacks, lack of concentration, loss of memory, disorientation, fits, convulsions, shock, addictions, frustration, irritability, aggression, violence, irrational behaviour, mood swings, delusions, hallucinations, nightmares, insomnia, anxiety, nervousness, tension, weeping, depression, lack of confidence, fears, clumsiness and inability to keep still.

Other symptoms which have been noted specifically in children are behavioural problems, hyperactivity, overexcitability, crying, rocking, retarded mental development, poor performance at school and speech and reading difficulties.

This wide range of mental symptoms can be due to food allergens, food additives or environmental pollutants, trace mineral deficiencies or toxic poisoning. Petrochemicals such as pesticides, insecticides, fertilisers, preservatives, and a whole range of potentially toxic substances, have all been incriminated in mental (and physical) illness. Remember, we are as much at risk from what we breathe as what we eat. Drugs of all types – including the contraceptive pill – can cause symptoms such as depression, and even allergy drugs can cause or aggravate mental symptoms.

The foods most often associated with mental illness are alcohol, milk, wheat and other grains, tea, coffee, sugar, chocolate, citrus fruits, eggs and cheese. Caffeine is well-known to cause anxiety, nervousness, irritability, palpitations and insomnia. Of the food additives, some artificial colourings, preservatives and flavourings are particularly bad. Also, there is some evidence that 620 L-glutamic acid and the sweetener aspartame (also known as *Nutrasweet* and *Canderel*) may affect the brain in susceptible people.

Recommended supplements are: vitamin C, 1–3g daily; B complex vitamins, vitamin E, zinc, magnesium and calcium. As patients who suffer from mental symptoms (allergy-induced or otherwise) may be lacking in essential fatty acids, a diet high in fish and oils such as soya, sunflower and olive are recommended.

See also **Behaviour Problems, Concentration (lack of), Confusion, Hearing Difficulties**, and **Hyperactivity**.

BREAST-FEEDING

Breast-feeding is a course of action and not a symptom, but it is so important that it justifies inclusion in this book. All the experts agree that breast-feeding is preferable to bottle-feeding. However, if you are one of those unfortunate people who just do not seem to be blessed with the ability to produce breast-milk, try not to feel too distressed. Look around you at all the bouncing children who have been entirely bottle-fed and put any guilty feelings out of your mind.

As a point of interest, the only clinical ecologist with whom I have discussed this subject told me that for mothers in this predicament he found that if he removed cow's milk from their diets, they were then able to produce breast-milk. In other words, it was his belief that such mothers were cow's milk-intolerant – an interesting theory and quite plausible in my opinion.

Breast-milk is the ideal food because it is of superior nutritional quality and, through it, the mother passes on antibodies to commonly found bacteria and viruses which protect her baby from infection – whereas formula feeding provides no such immunological protection against disease. This gives the baby a chance until he can start producing his own immunity. It also gives him the best potential for long-term mental and physical health.

Breast-feeding benefits all infants but particularly those from allergic backgrounds. For them, prolonged breast-feeding and careful weaning are the most important factors in diminishing the risks of developing allergies. Babies can be sensitised in the womb and, therefore, where there is a history of allergy on either side of the family, it is important for the mother to eat a well-balanced, varied diet of natural foods, with a limited intake of cow's milk, carefully avoiding any foods to which she knows herself to be sensitive. She should take extra calcium if she is on a milk-free diet. Alcohol should be kept to a minimum.

The prospective mother would be well advised to let the hospital know in advance that she wishes to breast-feed exclusively. The baby should *not* be given any sugar water on his first day. He should be put to the breast within hours of being born in order to benefit from the colostrum which precedes breast milk and which is high in nutrients. The mother should feed her baby on demand initially with a view to finding the schedule which best suits her and her baby. She will probably have to conform to the hospital routine to start with but when she returns home she can plan her own day. My advise is: listen to your own instinct. Every baby is different, every mother is different, every situation is different. You do what suits you and your baby best. Do not let anyone, however well intentioned, try to force their beliefs onto you. Ask advice by all means but do not necessarily feel obliged to follow it. Where your baby is concerned, *you* know best.

Try to breast-feed exclusively for three to six months. You will need a varied diet of fresh foods and plenty of fluids, and vitamin and mineral supplements will be very beneficial at this time. If you can resist introducing solids until he is six months old he is less likely to become sensitive to them. Also, it is advisable to leave those foods high in allergenic properties to last. Potential problem foods include cow's milk, eggs, wheat, fish and citrus fruits. *Never* give an infant or small child peanuts because, apart from the fact that they could easily stick in his throat, they are also potentially highly allergenic – and therefore dangerous.

The foods *least* likely to cause sensitivities are milk-free baby rice, puréed root vegetables, (potatoes, carrots, swede etc), pureed fruits (apple, pear, banana) followed by grain cereals (but not wheat), lamb, chicken and turkey. Introduce only one new food at a time (and only when your baby is well) and wean gradually over a period of months.

Whereas there is no doubt that 'breast is best', it can be, in cases of high sensitivity, a source of allergies because it carries proteins from the foods which the mother has eaten. If her baby develops a rash, colic or diarrhoea it could be because he is reacting to something she is eating which is passing through her breast milk. In this case, her best bet is to (temporarily) give up cow's milk (and its products) as this is the most likely cause and see if this will do the trick. If there is no improvement, she must try giving up the more potentially allergenic foods until she finds the culprit/culprits. (Never assume that a baby with diarrhoea, spots or colic is suffering from an allergy until your doctor has discounted infection. Any baby suffering from diarrhoea should be seen quickly as this type of infection can be very serious in infants and young children, as I know from personal experience.)

Where a mother cannot breast-feed, for whatever reason, she will be recommended a particular brand of baby formula with which, in the majority of cases, a strength will be found to suit her baby. Sometimes a different brand may prove more suitable. A minority of babies will not be able to tolerate cow's milk-based formulas as such, but in all likelihood they will be able to take *Pregestimil* or *Nutramigen* which are made from cow's milk but have been treated with digestive enzymes to break down their milk proteins. Alternatives for those babies who cannot tolerate a cow's milk-based feed in any shape or form are soya-based formulas such as *Formula S* or *Wysoy*. These contain no cow's milk whatsoever.

BREAST LUMPS

Every woman should examine her breasts regularly and if, at any time, she discovers a lump this should always be reported to her doctor. The great majority of breast lumps are benign and can even come and go. The doctor may arrange for her to have a mammogram and/or see a surgeon with a view to removing the lump to make certain it is not cancerous. Even in the minority of cases where a lump is found to be cancerous, treatment these days is much gentler, mastectomy (breast removal) being performed far less as other forms of treatment have developed.

However, it is worth considering that lumps can be caused by food sensitivity, although this fact should never stop you reporting a lump to your doctor. Caffeine and dairy products have both been reported but other foods could be responsible.

Professor Sir Richard Doll, head of the Imperial Cancer Research Fund Epidemiology Unit in Oxford and a world authority on cancer has warned that young women who take oral contraceptive pills for four or five years increase the risk of developing breast cancer. However, he is also quoted as saying that the results are open to different interpretations because the trials were done in the 1970s and the modern pills used nowadays are of a much lower dosage.

BREATHLESSNESS

Breathlessness can have a variety of causes, but the most common are respiratory infections and asthma. Breathlessness in asthma may be accompanied by a persistent cough and wheezing. Young children often wheeze with respiratory infections. Chronic smokers can become breathless and may develop a smoker's cough. Long-term smoking may lead to serious illness.

A doctor should be called in the following circumstances: if a baby is affected, if a foreign body is thought to be obstructing the air passages, if heart disease is involved, or if there is any obvious distress.

See also **Asthma** and **Bronchitis**.

BRONCHITIS

Bronchitis can be caused by a number of viruses and bacteria. It can also be caused by allergy. Very often it is a combination of several factors. It is a common condition frequently found in people living in a damp environment and in more polluted areas. Symptoms are a persistent cough, wheezing, breathlessness, phlegm which cannot be got rid of, and a general feeling of illness. It may or may not be accompanied by fever. If it is caused by infection, it is likely to last anything from seven to twenty-one days. It is advisable to contact the doctor as an antibiotic may be necessary, especially if the condition worsens or if it is accompanied by chest pain. A doctor should certainly be consulted where babies and the elderly are concerned as they are at greater risk of developing pneumonia.

Where bronchial attacks recur, environmental – rather than infective – agents should be considered. For example, there is a far higher than average incidence of bronchitis in people living near a gasworks or those who live in damp houses (or areas).

Asthma may be involved either by following an attack of bronchitis (it does not take much to trigger a susceptible person who is already wheezing) or by preceding it. When asthma causes the membranes lining the tubes in the lungs it becomes irritated, this provides an excellent environment for the germs which cause bronchitis, should the patient be exposed to them. From this it can be seen that the asthmatic is at greater risk. Hayfever, also, accompanied by a persistent cough, can develop into bronchitis if left untreated. This link with allergy is not always recognised.

Those people subject to bronchitis should avoid cold rooms, dust, fog, smokey atmospheres and open fires. Chemical fumes in even minute amounts can cause bronchitis in susceptible people. Other causes include air pollution, paint, gas, mould, damp and occupations which involve over-exposure to dusts or chemicals. Allergy to tobacco smoke and petrochemicals is also well documented and, of course, bronchitis can certainly be associated with a wide range of foods and/or food additives. Those additives which have been researched in connection with bronchitis are E102, E142, 621, 622 and 623. There are plenty more which may affect the individual.

Symptoms can be relieved by steam inhalations and by taking 3g of vitamin C daily and going down to a maintenance dose of 1g a day after recovery. Garlic perles and vitamins A and E are also said to be helpful. These can be taken in conjunction with an antibiotic without ill effects if one has been prescribed.

See also **Asthma** and **Breathlessness**.

BRUISING (SPONTANEOUS BRUISING OR PURPURA)

Spontaneous bruising, ie, bruising which has appeared without an external injury, can be caused by an infection or an allergic reaction to foods, drugs or chemicals (inhaled or ingested). Food additives are known to be responsible in some cases, E102 (tartrazine) being but one example. Spontaneous bruising is usually accompanied by other symptoms which may give a lead as to the most likely cause.

BULIMIA

Bulimia mostly affects adolescent girls. It is a condition which involves bouts of bingeing (ie, over-eating) followed by vomiting and a feeling of self-disgust. It is similar to anorexia but without the obsession to be constantly losing weight. There may be a strong craving for the foods on which the individual is bingeing. People who crave certain foods or drinks are addicted to them, and addiction and sensitivity go hand in hand. A sense of well-being often follows the consumption of a food to which someone is allergic. This sensation is inevitably followed by feeling low again and possibly other symptoms as well. Only the next 'fix' will right the situation. Food addiction, which may not always be the cause of bulimia, but most certainly is in some cases, resembles drug addiction and it is only too easy to understand how it can become habit forming. As with all such problems, however much parents or friends wish to help (and their encouragement is very valuable), in the end it comes down to the determination of the sufferer herself. Yes, you *can* overcome this if you really want to! Just keep trying and, if you slip up, don't worry but pick yourself up and start again. In the end you *will* succeed.

See also **Addiction** and **Anorexia Nervosa**.

BURPING

People have complained to me from time to time that continual burping has accompanied other symptoms in an allergic reaction. I can find no reference to this in any allergy books so obviously it is not a symptom often mentioned to the doctors. It seems that it can appear as a result of a reaction to either a food or an inhalant.

CANCER

Some doctors believe that allergies may be the forerunners of serious immune system disorders such as cancer. They say that prolonged exposure to an irritant or severe pressure on the immune system can impair the body's ability to check malignant cells.

My first comment is that allergies – certainly severe multiple allergies – are already indicative of an immune system disorder but one that can, in many cases, be stabilised if not rectified. My second point is that if cancer is caused by an immune system which is under-reacting (ie, allows the growth of unwanted cells) and those people who develop multiple allergies have an immune system which is over-reacting (ie, treats harmless matter as foreign) are we not, in fact, the opposite end of the spectrum?

When we talk about a 'miracle cure' in a cancer patient, we are referring to someone who was recognised as seriously (possibly terminally) ill but at some point, for no apparent reason, starts to recover. Whether or not we use the term miracle in its divine sense does not detract from the fact that there were physical reasons for this improvement but they are so complex that they probably went unrecognised.

In Britain we are very fortunate in having the Royal Marsden Hospital which caters for a large number of both inpatient and outpatient cancer sufferers. Although they would doubtless be reticent about using the term 'miracle cure', there is no doubt that some patients who have been given up as hopeless cases by other hospitals have made remarkable recoveries in their care. Other cancer centres have had their successes too. Therefore, highly skilled orthodox medical knowledge and treatment play a major part in many cases of unexpected recovery. However, to what extent can the patient play a part himself or herself? There is a school of thought which believes that visualising his cancer as the enemy and imagining his immune system marshalling its forces and leading them into successful combat is one step towards recovery. From this he will gain immense satisfaction that the cancer is being beaten and set all his bodily functions working *for* him, instead of against. The reversal of stress, in fact. This is a recognised form of therapy, known as visualisation, and has certainly worked for some people. However, I believe that it should be used as one factor in a recovery regime which involves a complete change of life-style. Other relevant factors are: plenty of fresh air and exercise, a well-regulated, healthy diet and a stress-free existence. This stress-free existence should include things which bring real pleasure, such as listening to music of your own choice and to programmes which will make you laugh – anything which will promote a sense of well-being in fact.

Accepting that heredity plays a major role, the general belief of orthodox *and* complementary medicine is that our western diet has a lot to answer for. Some doctors believe this to be the main cause of cancer and others believe that being exposed to external carcinogens (cancer-causing substances) over a period of time poses the greater threat. The different views are not so much between the orthodox doctors and the environmentalists as between individual doctors. There are those who are more interested in the various forms that cancer can take, and all the medical/scientific background that involves, and those who are interested in publicising the causes of cancer and thereby preventing it. We have reached common ground over smoking, and it would be a brave man indeed who would now say that he does not believe that the chemicals in tobacco are a major cause of lung cancer. Even here the individual's inherited susceptibility must not be overlooked. Otherwise, how have some people been able to survive being heavy smokers, escaping lung cancer and living to a ripe old age? Nevertheless, it is not a risk worth taking.

Sir Richard Doll, the eminent researcher who, with a colleague, established the connection between lung cancer and smoking in 1950, has stated his belief that western food, however, is an even greater underlying cause of cancer.

With regard to food-related cancers, there are several aspects to be considered. There is the belief that over-consumption of fats and sugars is relevant – as is under-consumption of fibre. (A lack of fibre will delay our bodies' natural functions, thereby allowing toxic matter to build up.) Over and over again in my research I have come across the common view that regularly eating over-refined, highly processed foods can cause cancer and yet such foods are not only permitted in bulk in our shops but are allowed to increase in number as every year goes by. Processed foods contain artificial additives and so-called 'natural' ones (which in fact, are not natural any more because they have been removed from their source of origin). It has been estimated that the people of Britain eat 6–15lb of additives on average per year. Premature deaths from cancer (also heart disease) are said to be higher in the UK than in any other European country. Are you surprised? People take coffee so much for granted that they probably do not think of it as a processed food. Yet it is. Dr Philip Cole reported in *The Lancet* a strong relationship between coffee consumption and cancer of the bladder and lower urinary tract.

The correct diet is vital to prevent cancers, and likewise is a necessary part of treatment for cancers also. Doctors Alec Forbes and Jan de Winter have pioneered this view and proved its success. So what *is* a wholesome diet which will help to keep us free from cancer (and, incidentally, a whole host of other diet-related diseases as well)? We need a high-fibre diet of 100% wholegrains, vegetables, fruit (raw as well as cooked) and extra bran for those who need to get things moving. We need to cut right down on the 'goodies' – cakes, biscuits, puddings, sweets, chocolates, alcohol and fizzy drinks. That makes life not worth living, you might argue. Strike a balance; only for those people who are suffering from cancer would I suggest a total restriction on these foods.

So, which are the food additives known or suspected of being carcinogenic? They are as follows: Yellow 2G, a yellow coal-tar dye similar to tartrazine; E123 amaranth, a red coal-tar dye, banned in the USA (this led to a ban on red 'Smarties' when they were imported from Britain); E153 Carbon Black, produced from burning plant material; E154 Brown FK, a synthetic mixture of azo dyes; E239 Hexamine, a synthetic derivative of benzene preservative; E249 potassium nitrite; E250 sodium nitrite; E251 sodium nitrate; E252 potassium nitrate. These last four are all preservatives. They react with amines to form nitrosamines which have been shown to be potentially carcinogenic. Nevertheless, without them pathogenic micro-organisms would grow in meats and would cause many deaths. E407 carrageenan is naturally extracted from seaweeds; only when it is degraded may it become carcinogenic. Other suspected additives are E231, E320, E321, E420(i), E420(ii), 430–436, 466, 621–623 and the sweeteners aspartame (also known as *Canderel* and *Nutrasweet)* and saccharin.

The 18 October 1989 issue of the *Daily Telegraph* stated 'Uniroyal, the American manufacturers of *Alar*, a pesticide used to promote the growth of apples and pears, is to withdraw the chemical worldwide for food use after public concern about its safety'. It went on to say that the decision followed earlier advice that *Alar* (or daminozide) was safe despite being withdrawn in America after scientists said that it might cause cancer. This decision came into being following the fears voiced by the UK Association, Parents for Safe Food. (Well done those parents, I say!) This is just one example of how the public have to *fight* for the right to have safe products.

'Every year two hundred million tons of potentially dangerous pollutants are released into the atmosphere.' So says Earl Mindell, author of *The Vitamin Bible.* He is of course referring to the USA, but we are equally guilty in Britain.

So what are all these pollutants? They come in the form of fumes from factories and power stations, fumes from car exhausts and all the multitude of other vehicles blocking our motorways, fumes from gas, oil and coal which we use in our homes and elsewhere, fumes from industry in general, and a wide range of chemicals we use in our homes and gardens. They come in the form of insecticides, pesticides, herbicides and artificial fertilizers, and last of all they come in the form of all the millions of pounds worth of scented toiletries we see fit to adorn ourselves with every year.

Skin cancer can be caused by over-exposure to the sun, especially in hot climates – which ours seems to be fast becoming. When in the hot sun it is advisable to expose the skin for just ten minutes the first day, building up the time gradually to allow the body to become acclimatised. Never fall asleep in the sun without someone around to rouse you as this can be dangerous. Fair-skinned people are more at risk than dark, and red-headed people particularly so.

Any chemical which causes prolonged irritation of the skin can, in time, cause skin cancer. Anyone who finds himself in this situation at work should seriously consider changing his job. Other cancers can be caused by inhaling chemicals, or some form of dust (asbestos, for example). It would be better if people stayed only a short time in jobs where they are at risk of such occupational hazards.

So, by now I have spoiled your pleasure in eating and drinking, your smoking, your romantic evenings and your sunbathing and got you worried about your job to boot! Well, let us put things into perspective. I have not given up these things (except smoking and additives), but hope that by striking a balance I will give myself a reasonable chance of not developing cancer. Should I be unfortunate enough to do so, I would make use of the best medical brains I could find, read all the books I could lay my hands on and find out all the means by which I could detoxify my body. Vitamins, A, C and E help to counteract the effects of toxins, and selenium is believed to contain properties which may neutralise certain carcinogens. I believe that no supplement can do you anything but good provided you do not exceed the recommended dose.

See aso **Breast Lumps**.

CANDIDIASIS

Candida albicans is one of the micro-organisms found in the gut of all human beings. The yeast-like fungus can multiply and cause infections or allergic reactions. An allergy to *Candida* is actually the liberation of *Candida* toxin. The condition is known as candidiasis or thrush. People who suffer from food or environmental allergies are particularly prone to it. However, even among doctors working in the field of environmental illness, there is some controversy as to the number of people who suffer from it. Some claim that the treatment of candidiasis leads to a great improvement in patients suffering from allergy. The theory is that, by reducing the load on the immune system, the development of further food sensitivities seems unlikely. A very logical argument. On the other hand, some people who have been diagnosed as candidiasis patients have later been proved to have had only straightforward food allergies. My own view is that, as the symptoms can be so similar, it is worth testing for food allergies first; this involves one to two weeks elimination diet prior to re-introduction, as opposed to going onto a 'candida diet' which involves dieting for two to three months.

Candidiasis can affect the skin, mouth, vagina or gut. On the skin it appears as a fungal-type rash in creases such as those between the toes. Oral thrush is a white plaque in the mouth and possibly a sore throat. Young and new born babies are particularly susceptible to this. Vaginal thrush produces a white vaginal discharge and itching. These forms of the condition are easily recognised. It is when candidiasis is found in the gut that it presents a greater problem of diagnosis. The symptoms may include bloating (distension of the abdomen), anal irritation, cystitis, indigestion, wind, abdominal pain, diarrhoea (or occasionally constipation) and sometimes symptoms such as depression as well. As already mentioned, these symptoms may be caused by other conditions also, including the equal likelihood of food allergy.

As there is no satisfactory diagnostic test, the doctor will have to be guided by the patient's medical and dietary history and, if the candida treatment is tried, by observation as to its success or otherwise.

This is a problem which has been highlighted only in the last couple of decades or so, and one of the reasons for this is the long-term use of broad-spectrum antibiotics. Recurrent or prolonged use of antibiotics kills off the good micro-organisms in the gut, thus allowing *Candida* to multiply freely. Another cause is the prolonged use of steroids, such as cortisone, which will suppress the immune system, thereby allowing *Candida* to flourish. The contraceptive pill is also a steroid, and so the same applies. This sort of hazard is never mentioned when women request the Pill – which I think is unforgivable because taking steroids long-term poses many potential hazards of which this is only one. Other stresses which suppress the immune system are vitamin deficiencies, viruses, emotional traumas and exposure to chemicals.

Another cause of *Candida* overgrowth is high sugar or yeast consumption or living in a mouldy environment. Depression and similar symptoms in candidiasis are caused by sensitivity to the person's own intestinal flora and will disappear as the treatment takes effect.

The most commonly used treatment is a course of nystatin – said to be a very safe drug – and a candida diet. The nystatin is usually taken orally as a powder. It destroys *Candida* without affecting the beneficial flora. Chemically-sensitive patients may notice an increase in symptoms over the first few weeks because, as the *Candida* die, the body may develop an allergic reaction to the organisms. This shows that the treatment is working. Some chemically-allergic people are not able to tolerate nystatin and will need to be desensitised first. There are alternative anti-*Candida* drugs; one is nizoral, but this is not so commonly used and is no good for the chemically sensitive.

A non-chemical approach is treatment with *Lactobacillus acidophilus*. This is a micro-organism which normally resides in the digestive tract. It is useful when other treatments cannot be tolerated. *L. acidophilus* is a form of good intestinal bacteria. (If doctors prescribed this or something similar in conjunction with antibiotics it could help to prevent the antibiotics destroying the good intestinal bacteria.) Taking it will help to restore the balance of the gut flora in the candida patient. One tablespoonful of 'acidophilus liquid' should be taken three times a day unless otherwise prescribed.

Oleic acid, which is found in cold-pressed olive oil, has been found to be helpful – as has yoghurt. Candida sufferers are often deficient in B vitamins – biotin especially – and 500mcg of the latter taken twice daily is recommended. A strong dose of B complex vitamins would be beneficial too.

Desensitisation to *Candida* can produce a rapid improvement, but as the neutralising level changes rather frequently this is not often considered practical.

The patient will, in addition, be recommended a sugar and yeast-free diet which will need to be continued for a matter of weeks, or possibly months; *do* persevere with the diet because many people have – eventually – improved dramatically in health as a result of doing so!

For Candida diet see page 26. See also **the Pill**.

CATARRH

Nasal catarrh can develop as either a direct or indirect result of colds or other infections involving the nose or sinuses. It can last for a few days to a few weeks. It can also be caused by allergy. Unfortunately, allergies lower resistance to infections, and infections make people more susceptible to allergies – so the cause may well be a combination of both.

Chronic catarrh may also be referred to as chronic sinusitis, repeated colds, post-nasal drip, round-the-year hay fever or perennial allergic rhinitis. Excess mucus from the nose trickles down the back of the throat and will either be swallowed or coughed up later.

Prolonged catarrh can lead to cough, sinusitis, congestion, wheezing and even bronchitis. Constant irritation of the nose and sinuses can lead to the growth of nasal polyps. Fortunately these are relatively rare and can be removed if they cause problems.

In chronic catarrh, mucus can accumulate in the eustachian tubes causing serous otitis or 'glue ear'. This can affect taste, smell and hearing. In fact it is one of the major causes of deafness in children. A vague, inattentive child may well turn out to be one who is unable to hear so it is advisable for all children to be given regular hearing tests. Any child suffering from serous otitis and left untreated could suffer permanent damage.

If catarrh is caused by a viral infection this can clear up gradually of its own accord. Nasal drops or sprays can ease the situation but should be taken only on a temporary basis they can accentuate the problem.

Seasonal catarrh has to be allergy-induced, and likely causes are tree, flower pollens or possibly moulds. The most common causes for all-year-round catarrh have been found to be foods, especially milk, wheat and eggs. Other foods implicated are citrus fruits, chocolate, beans, peas, tomatoes, potatoes, cheese, pork and oats. Even strong odours from cooking can cause catarrh in more sensitive people. Chemicals can also be responsible or, at least, aggravate the situation. Catarrh will be made worse by exposure to car exhaust and other fumes, dust, tobacco smoke, paint, gas and changes in temperature. Excessive use of decongestant nose drops can cause catarrh.

The most important thing to do, as with all allergic reactions, is to find the cause. If this turns out to be seasonal, and therefore unavoidable, then antihistamines certainly have their uses. Many people over-use these useful drugs so if you can cut down it is wise to use the smallest effective dose. Be wary of steroids. Prolonged use of steroids can be dangerous and produce unwanted side-effects. Some people prefer homeopathic treatments. Another alternative is saline drops (one-quarter teaspoonful of salt in a tumbler of warm water) which, if inserted into each nostril daily, can bring relief. Some people claim that a vitamin A supplement is effective.

See also **Hay Fever** and **Sinusitis**.

CHEST PAINS

Chest pains may have a serious cause so a doctor should always be consulted, especially where a heart condition is already known or suspected or if the pain is accompanied by pallor and sweating.

Chest pains which are a symptom of a disorder of the heart such as angina, may be brought on by exercise, particularly climbing. Even ascending the stairs may be sufficient to cause them. Sometimes the same pain is noticed after eating, especially a heavy meal, and may extend to shoulders and arms as well. With other people the pain may seem to be unrelated to any activity. In most instances, rest and pain-killers will alleviate the pain.

It is not always recognised that, as well as the blood vessels, the heart itself can also react allergically to both food and chemical allergens. Sometimes quite severe symptoms are involved – such as anginal pain, palpitations and even the closure of one of the heart's blood vessels. These symptoms may be accompanied by others, such as nausea, nervousness, shaking, insomnia, sweating and loss of weight.

The most common cause for allergy-induced chest pains – whether on the left- or right-hand side – is caffeine-containing foods and drinks, namely coffee, tea, chocolate and cola. Some people bring the problem on themselves by taking caffeine in excess, usually in the form of coffee. (Over five cups a day is positively not recommended for anyone.) Other people have become so sensitised that they react to very small amounts – although it may be to the particular drink that they are sensitive rather than the caffeine. Coffee is the most common and probably the most addictive, with tea coming a close second.

Other foods which have been found to cause chest pains include eggs, fish, shellfish, pork and food colourings.

See also **Angina** and **Heart Conditions**.

CHOKING

Choking may be due to inhaling a foreign substance. In an allergic reaction, choking due to swelling of the tongue or throat can block the windpipe and cause unconsciousness. Immediate medical attention is required to enable the patient to breathe again. If he begins to turn blue, take the handle of a spoon and gently press down the patient's tongue in order to allow air to pass into the windpipe while waiting for help.

Such violent reactions can be caused by certain foods such as eggs, peanuts and shellfish. Pencillin-derived antibiotics can also be responsible, as can wasp and bee stings.

See also **Anaphylactic Shock**.

CLAUSTROPHOBIA

Claustrophobia means a fear of being in a crowded place with not much room to move, and it includes being shut up in small places such as lifts etc. Of course, this phobia can be readily understood in people who have suffered from some frightening experience in such circumstances. In fact, the majority of people who suffer from claustrophobia have not. So what causes people to develop this very real fear? Allergy of the brain is one cause. There may well be others of a psychological nature. Only people who have experienced allergies affecting the brain can really understand that sudden feeling of panic which descends out of the blue whilst waiting in a supermarket queue or equally crowded place. You have to get out and away and be on your own, preferably back in your own home *there and then.*

For some people the reaction will come on suddenly and unexpectedly; others will be bogged down on a continual basis, depending on how often they come into contact with the allergen which is affecting them.

Common causes are coffee, tea, milk, wheat, corn, chemical additives and a whole host of inhalant chemicals.

See also **Agoraphobia**.

COELIAC DISEASE

The tendency to develop coeliac disease is inherited and, in the more severe cases, is likely to be diagnosed in infancy. Less obvious cases with less specific symptoms may go undetected for years. Coeliac disease is the inability to tolerate gluten, one of the major proteins found in wheat, barley, rye and oats; therefore, it does not become apparent until the infant is weaned onto one – or a combination – of these grains.

Prior to diagnosis, the baby or child will fail to thrive, its muscles will become wasted, its abdomen distended and it will produce pale, soft, smelly motions which float. Vomiting can occur, and the child may become anaemic. As these symptoms can be caused by other conditions it is necessary to have the diagnosis confirmed by a special test which involves taking a biopsy of the lining of the bowel. If the diagnosis is confirmed, and gluten is removed from the diet, the child's health should return to normal. Thus, the symptoms can be stabilised but, in the great majority of cases, gluten must always be avoided as the condition is life-long. (Only if the condition is diagnosed very early in life is there a chance of it being reversible). However, the earlier gluten is introduced into an infant's diet the higher the chances appear to be of developing coeliac disease, a principle which applies to all food intolerances. Delaying the introduction of all solids for as long as possible, therefore, gives your child's digestive and immune systems a chance to mature.

Coeliac disease is more prevalent in children who have a family history of relatives with other allergy-induced illnesses. That those children who suffer from coeliac disease are more likely to produce other food and chemical sensitivities is indisputable. Robert Eagle, author of *Eating and Allergy*, shows the reverse side of the coin by stating that one child in ten who already suffers from milk allergy in infancy will go on to develop coeliac disease.

Coeliacs must stick conscientiously to a gluten-free diet because when gluten is eaten it causes damage to the lower bowel lining so that other foods cannot be properly absorbed. This means that other proteins will be inadequately digested, thus causing further intolerances. (Why the medical profession is able to accept the fact of a gluten-intolerance but cannot apply the same principle to other proteins is an anomaly it seems quite unable to explain.)

So if your child has some or all of these symptoms but his test comes back negative, and the medical profession has assured you that no other disease process is involved, what do you do? Consider other food allergies – including even wheat-sensitivity (which is quite different from gluten-sensitivity and would not show up in a coeliac test). Put him onto an elimination diet (see Introduction) in order to detect the food or foods to which he may be reacting.

What if your child shows a positive result to his test but his symptoms do not totally clear on a gluten-free diet? In this case there are two possibilities to consider. He may also be suffering from other undetected food or chemical allergies, which an elimination diet should expose. The second point is that some gluten-free products (which are available on prescription) still contain small traces of gluten, and these may be sufficient to produce his symptoms. Medicines as well as starch-containing products can be a source of gluten. Wheat is a cheap commodity and is frequently used as a filler. Watch out for ingredients listed as 'edible starch', 'cereal filler', 'cereal binder' and 'cereal protein'. They, as well as 'wheat starch', may be made from wheat also.

Although some people may be able to get away with small amounts of gluten occasionally, others, more severely afflicted, will not. For them, home-made products are much safer. A wide variety of gluten-free flours is available from health food shops. These include soya flour, rice flour, cornflour, pea flour, maize flour and others. Varying the choice of flours lessens the chances of developing further sensitivities.

Coeliacs, as with other allergy sufferers, can benefit by taking vitamin and mineral supplements.

COLIC

Colic is the term used to describe tummy pains suffered by some young babies. These cause them to cry out, go red in the face, draw up their legs and pass a lot of wind. I imagine it is comparable to a rather nasty bout of indigestion in adults. This tends to happen more often in the evenings.

The general belief is that colic begins around three weeks of age and will affect a baby for about three months. In fact a baby can suffer from colic from birth and can last much longer than three months, depending on the baby, the severity of the condition and what is done about it.

If a hitherto contented baby begins to scream in obvious pain, the doctor should be contacted right away. In rare cases it could be due to an obstruction in the intestines. In fact, all babies suffering from colic-type symptoms should be seen by a doctor in order to eliminate any other serious problems.

It having been established that your baby is 'only suffering from colic', what should you do about it? Well, you need to discover the cause, because, believe me, there is a cause. Doing this will save him and you weeks (or months) of unnecessary stress. Babies who suffer from colic which goes unchecked are more likely to develop eczema or asthma at a later stage than those whose allergens are discovered and removed.

The major cause of colic is an allergy to cow's milk which is a good reason for breast-feeding and not permitting anyone to give him complementary feeds whilst in hospital. A baby can be sensitised in the womb and born with a ready-made intolerance, or colic may start shortly after he is first bottle-fed or when he is weaned onto cow's milk. The more sensitive infant can even react to the cow's milk protein which passes through the mother's breast milk to her baby.

If you are breast-feeding him and have already introduced solids, cut these out for a day or two. It may be that he is allergic to one of them. In this case, the colic will soon disappear and you can test him on each food individually to see which is the culprit. If you are breast-feeding him but have not yet introduced solids (which is more likely) it may be that he is reacting to something *you* are consuming. Try removing cow's milk from your diet first. This will necessitate temporarily removing *all* cow's milk products too. Again, you should see an improvement within a few days if you have struck lucky. Otherwise you will have to try giving up a few foods at a time until you find out which is causing his problems.

Among the most common offenders are wheat, alcohol, tea, coffee, cheese, eggs, fish, shellfish, chocolate, nuts, peanuts, citrus fruits, yeast and artificial additives. In rare cases it may be nothing to do with allergy but may be simply that he is getting too much breast milk which he is not able to digest properly. However, this is uncommon.

If you are bottle-feeding him, check that the hole in the teat is the right size. If it is too large he will be getting too much milk too quickly, which would be responsible for his colic. An intake of air will do the same if the hole is too small.

If you have just weaned him from the breast, then it looks as if the milk you have chosen is not suiting him. Changing to another brand may be the answer for a few babies, but for the majority a different *type* of milk will be necessary.

Alternatives to cow's milk-based formulas are *Pregestimil* and *Nutramigen* which do contain cow's milk but have been treated with digestive enzymes which lessen their allergenic properties thereby making them more easily tolerated. Other alternatives are soya-based products such as *Prosobee*, *Wysoy* and *Formula S*. They contain no cow's milk; they are chemically similar to breast milk and are made from the soya bean to which vitamins, minerals and iron have been added.

Babies suffering from colic due to lactose intolerance (which means that they are deficient in the enzyme lactase required to digest the lactose present in milk) will need to be put onto one of the soya-based milks which are lactose-free.

A very few babies cannot tolerate even the soya baby milks. This is rare but should you find it applies to your baby, do not despair. Babies can thrive very well without any form of milk (and there are plenty around to tell the tale) but you will need expert advice so I suggest you visit a dietitian. This can be arranged through your doctor either on the NHS or privately if you so choose.

How can you best help a baby in the throes of colic? Hold him over your shoulder and pat him or rock him. If this does not pacify him, the rhythm of a walk in his pram or a drive in the car may help. If going out is not convenient, just walking gently around a room with him in your arms will soothe him, though it may take time. Try to avoid colic medications: they can sometimes affect the gut and, as often as not, contain artificial colourings and other additives. One of the most effective and least harmful products is gripe water, which, for years, has been used satisfactorily to alleviate colic in babies. I suggest that you avoid all unnecessary medications for your baby anyway – and for yourself, especially if breast-feeding.

Remember that babies cry because this is their only means of communication. They *need* to tell you if they are cold, uncomfortable, hungry or ill. If your instinct tells you that your baby needs you, go to him and ignore the experts who tell you it is natural for babies to cry. Most 'experts' have not brought up colicky babies; many are not even parents, let alone mothers, who have most exposure to their babies' distress.

The most contented babies are likely to be those who are exclusively breast-fed for four, preferably six months or longer. If you can delay introducing solids until this stage it will give your baby's digestive and immune systems time to mature so that he is better able to tolerate new foods.

If you are one of those unfortunate people (as I was) who very much want to breast-feed but find that no milk is forthcoming, let me assure you that it is quite possible to rear healthy babies in spite of this. It is possible that some women do not produce breast milk because they have a cow's milk allergy themselves which they have not recognised. By removing cow's milk from their diets, it may well reverse the situation. They could then find that they are doing themselves a favour as well as their baby! Keep trying and good luck to you! If all else fails, remember: he *will* grow out of it!

CONCENTRATION, LACK OF

Lack of concentration occurs mostly when a person has something on his mind which is worrying him – tension and anxiety add to the problem and it becomes even harder to concentrate. Overwork, tiredness and poor health are other common factors involved. Apparent lack of concentration in children frequently turns out to be due to poor hearing. Obviously, there are many possible causes and it is essential to find out where a child is concerned as he will have no insight into his state or the reasons for it himself.

One possibility which must be considered is allergies which effect the brain. Any allergy suffered to a sufficient degree is likely to involve the brain. Anyone who suffers badly from hay fever will confirm this. Many an allergic child has difficulty in concentrating at school for this reason. Also, there are allergic people whose specific target area is the brain just as in others it may be the skin, joints or gut. If affected badly enough they will have difficulty in assimilating even the simplest of facts.

Any foods, food additives or inhalants can be responsible. People usually react very promptly to exposure to chemicals which are inhaled, whereas food allergy reactions are more likely to be delayed.

All allergic people benefit from taking vitamins and mineral supplements, and it is thought that vitamin B12 and certain amino acids may help here.

See also **Brain Allergies, Hypoglycaemia.**

CONFUSION

One tends to think in terms of the elderly in relation to confusion and of course it is the main symptom of senile and pre-senile dementia. In fact there are many elderly people whose minds are very clear to a ripe old age.

Other reasons for confusion are the effects of drink or drugs, severe stress or fatigue, head injuries which may or may not involve concussion, a high fever, the after-effects of an epileptic fit or a stroke. There can be other serious causes so, if in doubt, consult a doctor. Confusion can also be caused by allergic reactions.

When referred to in medical documents, confusion and other mental symptoms are usually simply stated as facts as related by the onlooker. I hope to give insight into what the confused person is experiencing.

The confused person is unable to assimilate all but the simplest of facts, perhaps not even these. To get through the day without disaster requires the utmost concentration. Conversations mean nothing, but some form of response is required – one just hopes that it is the right one! The confused person sees without perceiving because he cannot absorb what he sees. Names are jumbled or forgotten. People look familiar but you do not remember who they are. It is not even possible to explain what is the matter because the words you require are not there. If you are old I imagine that you feel people will excuse you. If you are not old and have commitments and obligations, and possibly a job, the experience is frightening and humiliating and not many people are going to understand! Any of the common foods or chemical inhalants can be responsible.

See also **Brain Allergies, Hypoglycaemia.**

CONJUNCTIVITIS

When the conjunctiva become inflamed the eyes will be sore and red and possibly sticky. They will be worse first thing in the morning. If there is associated pain, it is important to see your doctor at once in the rare possibility that there is a serious underlying illness.

Mostly, however, the cause is either a viral or a bacterial infection, or else it is due to an allergy. In the case of the former it is very contagious but with medical treatment should clear up fairly quickly.

Allergic conjunctivitis falls into two categories: that which is caused by extreme sensitivities to things such as cosmetics, proprietary eye preparations, tobacco smoke or chemicals, and those types caused from within by foods or by food additives such as artificial colourings.

Whatever the cause, the eyes can be bathed in warm water; if they have not recovered within a few days, consult your doctor. If the condition does not clear up with eye drops or ointment then a swab may be taken. Should this test come back negative, and the condition persist, the likelihood is that it is caused by sensitivity of one kind or another.

The most common form of allergic conjunctivitis, however, is accompanied by rhinitis or respiratory complaints, as in hay fever. In this case, the eyes will be red, watery and not sore but itchy. This is probably due to grass, tree or flower pollen. If it is all the year round it will be due to a constant source of allergen such as house-dust mite, tobacco smoke, animal dander, house-plants or some chemicals in your environment.

Occasionally, conjunctivitis can be caused by cosmetics, proprietary eye washes, or even carelessness when spraying perfume or hair spray. The eyes can swell, and blurred vision may be experienced.

The best treatment for any form of allergic conjunctivitis is *Opticrom*, which is sodium cromoglycate in the form of eye drops. It has a good safety record and few side-effects.

Remember, *sore* eyes are most likely to have an infective cause, and *itchy* eyes are more likely to be due to an allergy.

Vitamins A and D, and those of the B complex, are said to be of value for people susceptible to this condition.

CONSTIPATION

C

Suffering from constipation does not mean passing stools less frequently – this in itself is of no great importance. It is the formation of the stools and the discomfort factor which are relevant, as is the feeling of wanting to go and not being able to. Small, hard, uncomfortable stools which are difficult to pass have a concentrated toxic content and therein lies the danger. Constipation is not uncommon during pregnancy, and your doctor will advise if this happens.

Caroline Walker and Geoffrey Cannon, co-authors of *The Food Scandal* say: 'We are a constipated nation. Almost one in five British people take laxatives.' They go on to say: 'It is thought that by increasing the bulk of stools and speeding up the flow through the lower gut and the bowel, fibre exercises the intestines, reduces pressure, prevents straining at stool and dilutes the waste matters in stools that are potential causes of cancer.'

Other disorders associated with constipation, apart from cancer, are diverticulitis, piles, intestinal polyps and possibly appendicitis. Constipation can, in itself, be a symptom of more complex conditions such as ulcerative colitis.

It is best to seek medical advice if the problem persists, if it does not respond to your own treatment, or if abdominal pain is present. Your doctor will advise on diet. He may prescribe laxatives which should be used only as a temporary measure. Constipation can be worsened by the over-use of laxatives as the patient becomes more dependent on them. Also, they tend to rob the body of essential nutrients. Enemas will rarely be necessary. For babies with constipation an increased amount of sugar in their feed will help to loosen their motions.

The causes of constipation are a lack of fibre (roughage) in the diet, a lack of fluids, or just too little food. (A few more serious conditions may cause constipation – hypothroidism, for example, but then other symptoms are always present which would point to a diagnosis.) Constipation may occur if we go somewhere other than our own home. There may be a psychological or an environmental reason for this. Either way, it will probably right itself within a short time.

If you are this way inclined, is there much you can do about it? There is indeed! This is the classic example of the patient's fate being in his own hands. Drinking water helps to prevent constipation – take plenty! Increase your intake of other fluids also. A diet containing plenty of roughage is the best prevention of constipation. So, which foods contain roughage? Wholegrains (grains in their unrefined state) – wheat, barley, oats, rye and corn (also known as maize). Wholemeal bread and wholemeal flour and bran also come into this category, as do vegetables (especially good are peas, beans and lentils) and fruit (especially good are figs and prunes). All vegetables contain fibre and, for those who prefer it, soup can be made from blended vegetables to which stock has been added. Bran flakes and bran tablets are useful, but do not overdo the bran at the expense of other forms of fibre.

For those people who suffer from food sensitivities and may not be able to tolerate the above grains, they can get their fibre from pulses, brown rice, buckwheat, millet, soy and rice bran. Taking a diet high in fibre not only speeds up the natural processes but also helps to prevent the build-up of toxic chemicals in the intestines and colon.

The same principles apply to everyone, but allergic people may have the added problem that a certain food (or foods) may cause constipation – a food which does not cause this in others. Like all allergic reactions, this will be an individual one; it will probably be a food commonly taken, and could even be one of those mentioned as having the opposite effect on everyone else – such is the lot of the allergy sufferer!

For those few people for whom the above advice does not seem to produce the desired effect, a bulk laxative such as *Isogel* or *Normacol* may be required. These are made from the husks of plant seeds so they should be tolerated by most food allergics. Other recommendations are the regular use of *Lactobacilus acidophilus*, an acidophilus culture, to keep the intestines clean (one tablespoon taken three times daily), kelp, bran tablets and a good preparation of B complex vitamins.

Never give a laxative to anyone with a bad stomach pain (especially a child) without specific advice from a doctor, because if this turned out to be appendicitis it could be dangerous.

See also **Irritable Bowel Syndrome** and **Ulcerative Colitis**.

CONVULSIONS (FITS)

Convulsions can occur in young children when there is a rapid rise in temperature at the onset of, or during, an illness. This is more likely to happen in the late afternoon or evening. The child looks blank, stiffens and then his limbs begin to twitch, sometimes quite violently. His eyes will turn upwards and he may go blue. It is a very frightening experience for the onlooker (and also, presumably, the child) but do try to remain calm. The fit will last for a matter of minutes, to be followed by a deep sleep usually lasting several hours. These are known as febrile convulsions and most children will have outgrown them by the age of five.

To prevent a child developing a febrile convulsion if he is already known to be unwell, try to reduce his temperature by keeping him cool. This can be done by removing some of his clothing and bedclothes, opening the windows, sponging him down with tepid water and giving him drinks. (It may all happen too quickly for you to have time to do any of this.) Ask your doctor whether he would advise an anti-convulsant drug to use as a preventative.

In a febrile convulsion (or indeed any type of fit), lay the child on his side with plenty of space around him, loosen his collar, and do not try to restrict his movements. A clean, rolled-up hanky or a metal spoon can be pushed between his teeth (if this is possible) to prevent injury to his tongue. A doctor should always be called for when a child has a convulsion.

Dr Paul Carson, in his book *How to Cope with your Child's Allergies*, says 'Recent research has shown that certain foods can provoke both high temperatures and convulsions in those children who are susceptible'. Neither he nor anyone else gives any indication as to specific foods which might be incriminated, but those listed under the entry 'Epilepsy' might be worth considering. Certainly food additives may be responsible.

Whilst I believe that this piece of research is very valuable, one must remember that many children are prone to infections, and when their temperature rises rapidly they run the risk of having a convulsion.

See also **Epilepsy**.

CO-ORDINATION, LACK OF

Lack of co-ordination may be due to ataxia, a symptom of many different diseases affecting the brain, where the patient has difficulty with movement and balance. Cerebral palsy, or spasticity, indicates a disorder of the brain present from birth which affects movement and co-ordination. Obviously, an early diagnosis is essential in either case.

Lack of co-ordination can also be due to an allergy which affects the brain. There is very little written in isolation on this aspect of allergic reaction but there is no doubt that many people known to be allergic have found their co-ordination to be affected after eating or inhaling a known allergen. (Chemical inhalants can be responsible, as can foods, depending on the individual response.)

One of my own experiences when affected this way is that I become unable to return a table-tennis ball to the other side of the table whereas normally I play quite a reasonable game! Another recognised result of this symptom is a quite obvious deterioration in handwriting. This has been observed in hyperactive children, for example. Clumsiness and other symptoms showing a degeneration in co-ordination are often present also.

As this symptom is frequently caused by certain food additives in susceptible people, it could easily disappear when junk food is replaced by a good, wholesome diet.

COT DEATHS

It is said that one in five hundred babies under six months old dies whilst asleep. The medical profession at large says there is no known cause.

COT DEATHS

Research led by Dr Kevin Forsyth, a lecturer in Paediatrics and Immunology at Flinders University in South Australia, turned up some interesting findings whilst he was working at the Institute of Child Health at London University. The study, published in the British Medical Journal, found higher levels of immunoglobulin in the lungs of infants who have died of cot deaths. The changed levels may be the result of trivial infections attacking the child at risk, apparently. (Could the 'child at risk' be the child who is also more susceptible to allergic responses, one wonders?) The evidence suggested that the respiratory tract was the prime target organ. Dr Forsyth suggested that these trials paved the way for further investigation.

I should like to put a hypothesis to you. In fact it is not so much a hypothesis as a series of known and accepted, medically proven facts.

Babies can be sensitised to food prior to birth by food molecules carried by the mother's blood into the baby's blood stream. After he is born, the baby can become sensitised also to the foods and drinks his mother takes, via her breast-milk, albeit in a more dilute form. He can, alternatively or in addition, become sensitised from his own *first* intake of food, producing anti-bodies which will cause a reaction the *second* time that food is taken.

Babies are particularly vulnerable to allergic reactions because allergy is a condition involving the immune system and their immune systems are very immature. Allergic reactions can come on rapidly, be severe, disappear, and leave no symptoms in their wake. If swelling of the tongue, mouth or airways is involved, then a baby (or anyone else for that matter) can die of suffocation. Severe allergic reactions can lead to anaphylactic shock, which is a form of collapse which can prove fatal.

Some research has been done into allergy being a possible cause of cot deaths. The idea that cot deaths might be due to allergy to cow's milk was propounded in the 1960s. Interest was lost in this hypothesis when it was realised that totally breast-fed babies died from cot deaths too. Even if it were not realised then that breast-fed babies could react to foods ingested by their mothers, one wonders why an intolerance to other foods was not considered alongside the cow's milk allergy theory.

Long ago, I knew personally two people whose babies had to be rushed to hospital by ambulance for emergency treatment because their lives were threatened. One baby had reacted to her first taste of egg yolk and was rapidly going blue in the face. The other, an older one, had eaten a grape and was reacting in the same way. The lives of these children were saved because the allergic responses were fairly rapid, the mothers reacted quickly, and medical treatment was prompt. What if the reactions had been delayed as they so often can be? Might not the child have been put to bed and left undisturbed to sleep?

I am not suggesting that allergy is the only cause of cot deaths – of course there must be others – but I am suggesting that it may not be uncommon. That being so, the best way to avoid the risk of a cot death (and incidentally lessen the risk of your baby developing allergies in general) is by the following means. Breast-feed for a minimum of four to six months, longer if you can. Take a wide and varied diet of fresh foods yourself, drink plenty (water preferably) and take a good vitamin and mineral supplement (without artificial additives) and be prepared to give frequent feeds. One gramme of vitamin C daily (taken by you) will help to protect your baby from being a cot death victim.

The longer you can delay giving him solids the better able his digestive and immune systems will be to cope with them. Introduce only one food at a time until you are sure that he can take it without adverse effect, and only give him a new food when he is well. Try him on the least allergenic foods first. Start with pureed root vegetables, including potatoes. Pureed fruit should be all right too (but leave the citrus fruits until later). Other vegetables and cereals (excluding wheat) come next. Baby rice which is milk-free is fine; you can mix this with water or expressed milk. Then try minced lamb, turkey, chicken and beef. Leave fish, eggs, wheat, citrus fruits, cow's milk and its products until the end of his first year. Check for reactions whenever a new food is introduced, especially when weaning onto cow's milk. In families where there is a history of allergy, a soya-based formula may be the best choice.

In taking these precautions, the chances are you will have a happy, contented baby who will thrive well.

See also **Colic**.

COUGHS

Coughing is symptomatic of many different diseases, including numerous infections of the cold/'flu variety. The cough may persist for some time after the other symptoms have vanished. It is not in its way a bad thing as it is the body's way of ridding the lungs of irritants. However, it is annoying and can be very exhausting if it persists.

If infection is not the cause then a sensitivity probably exists. In a few cases this may be related to occupation, especially if dust particles or chemicals are involved. Once a cough (or any other symptom for that matter) develops in these circumstances then it is essential to get away from the source of contact.

Coughing can be an early symptom of either asthma or hay fever and, in mild cases, may be the main or only symptom, possibly with throat-clearing as well. (Some people cough only at night or on exertion.) On the other hand it may be accompanied by runny eyes and nose, and sneezing, in the case of hay fever, or breathing difficulties or wheezing in the case of asthma. It is the main symptom of bronchitis when the patient may have a fever also.

Causes are numerous – pollens, house dust and chemical sensitivities being some of the main ones. Bronchitis is as likely to be caused by an infection as an allergy.

Beware of patent cough medicines. They often contain all sorts of chemicals, including chemical additives, to which the patient may be sensitive. In any case they are unlikely to be of much benefit. My own remedy is half a squeezed lemon, two teaspoonfuls of honey and one teaspoonful of glycerine in a mug of hot water, but any warm drink will be equally soothing. One gramme of vitamin C daily will help to ease the cough, whatever the cause.

See also **Asthma, Bronchitis, Croup** and **Hay Fever**.

CRAMP

Cramp is a contraction of a muscle or muscles. It happens suddenly and quite involuntarily and causes acute pain. People with poor muscular co-ordination are prone to it. Sportsmen, especially swimmers, may suffer from it. Any constant use of the same muscles may lead to cramp. Writer's cramp, for example, is brought on by constant writing.

Bowel or stomach cramps are often associated with diarrhoea. Some people are more likely to suffer at night. Cramps of all kinds can be caused by allergies, most likely to foods; another cause is lack of salt.

Sportsmen who play energetic sports lose a lot of salt in sweating; this is why they are prone to cramps. They can take extra salt either as a precaution or when they actually develop cramp; this will give immediate relief.

As all sufferers are said to be short of sodium and chlorine, they will all benefit from increasing their salt intake unless they suffer from hypertension or any other condition where this could be dangerous. The B vitamins and vitamin D are also recommended.

CROHN'S DISEASE (REGIONAL ILEITIS)

In Crohn's disease the lower part of the small bowel, and possibly other parts of the digestive tract, become inflamed. The wall of the intestine thickens, and ulcers and infection develop. Diarrhoea, fever and weight loss occur, and there is abdominal pain which can become very severe. Complications may result, and other different types of symptoms flare up. This disease is also known as ileitis. It affects mostly young Jewish adults. Some people will suffer only one or a few random attacks whereas for others it will be a life-long condition.

After sending the patient to hospital for tests to confirm the diagnosis, the doctor will prescribe drugs to combat the diarrhoea and possibly a short course of steroids in severe cases. If there are complications he may suggest an operation but this is no guarantee that the condition will improve.

There is little doubt that these symptoms are related to the ingestion of certain foods but it is not yet known whether this is due to food intolerance or to an enzyme deficiency. Either way, discovering the foods involved (differing in the individual) and removing them from the diet will usually lead to a recovery in people suffering from Crohn's disease. Dr Jonathan Brostoff, in his excellent book *The Complete Guide to Food Allergy and Intolerance*, writing of Dr John Hunter of Addenbrooke's Hospital, Cambridge, says: 'He finds that over eighty per cent of patients recover on an elimination diet and then react to specific foods when these are reintroduced. By cutting out the incriminated foods, these patients remain well.' Crohn's disease patients are very ill, and carrying out an elimination diet can be hazardous; Dr Brostoff recommends that 'If you have Crohn's disease, you should not consider trying an elimination diet without full medical supervision.' However, this is not always easy to come by, so trying to eliminate one or two of the most likely foods at a time might just throw some light on the problem. Dr Brostoff says that patients take about nine days, on average, to respond, but could take more than two weeks in some cases.

There is no record to show which foods are more likely to be responsible, but as the main symptoms are diarrhoea and abdominal pain it could be that the foods which are known to be the most likely to cause these symptoms in isolation would be worth considering first.

As this is such a debilitating disease, all sufferers will benefit from taking 1g of vitamin C daily, a good strong preparation of B complex vitamins and a good multi-mineral. Acidophilus culture (a source of friendly intestinal bacteria) can work wonders for people suffering from diarrhoea – three capsules or two tablespoonfuls of the liquid should be taken three times a day.

See also **Abdominal Pain** and **Diarrhoea**.

CROUP

Croup is a condition affecting the larynx of children under the age of five and mostly in the first two years of life. It can come on suddenly and cause a hoarse, barking cough which can give you quite a shock the first time you hear it. It is accompanied by noisy breathing and a fever. If you are concerned, call the doctor and certainly call him if any of the following apply: the child has a high temperature, has difficulty in breathing, says that his throat hurts, cannot swallow, or looks pale.

Most cases are not as serious as they would seem, and the child makes a quick recovery. Give him plenty of cool drinks. Boil a kettleful of water in a small room which will soon fill with steam and reassure your child as he sits on your knee. This atmosphere will help to overcome the worst of his croup and he should improve quite quickly.

Although croup is commonly considered an infectious viral disease, there is a belief that, in some cases, *recurrent* croup may be caused by an allergy. No foods have been researched in this respect but bear in mind that milk, wheat and eggs are the most common offenders in general terms, and artificial additives are suspect in all complaints. In susceptible children a chemical inhalant, such as smoking, may be enough to trigger an attack. A good multi-vitamin to help build up resistance to both infections and allergies is *Junamac* (*mini-Junamac* for babies after weaning), marketed by Cantassium Co Ltd.

CYSTITIS

Cystitis is inflammation of the bladder. It is most common in newly married and pregnant women and is uncommon in men and children. A full investigation should be carried out where a child is concerned to ensure that the kidney tubes are free from infection.

Acute cystitis lasts for about five days and is usually caused by a bacterial infection. The chronic form can last for long periods if left untreated. There is severe pain and frequency of urination (not to be confused with frequent urination *without* pain – see Enuresis). Pain in the lower abdomen and cloudy urine are common, and there may be a rise in temperature. The most usual causes are infection following sexual intercourse or a germ from the bowel. Much less usual is some congenital abnormality.

If symptoms persist for more than a day or two, consult your doctor. He should be consulted immediately if the symptoms are severe or if there is blood in the urine. He may carry out a vaginal examination (rectal in men) or prescribe antibiotics or both. Occasionally he will recommend a hospital visit to exclude other underlying causes. He will certainly advise an increase in fluid intake – at least five pints a day is recommended in whatever form you wish (don't overdo the caffeine!). Water is best, however, and lemon barley water is good too. (People who do not want to take the processed one can make their own by boiling up barley, extracting the water, and adding lemon and sugar, or honey. Take pain-killers for a limited time if necessary, and always complete a prescribed course of antibiotics. One tablespoonful of potassium citrate mixture (obtainable from your chemist) in half a glass of water taken three times a day will help to clear the symptoms.

To prevent a recurrence, women are advised to take plenty of baths, avoid constipation, avoid going for long periods without liquids, and always go to the lavatory after intercourse has taken place. Some women may need to avoid using scented toiletries.

Recurrent cystitis which is not due to bacterial infection is likely to be due to an allergy. This could be a reaction to rubber or chemical contraceptives or to bath products, deodorants or other vaginal toiletries.

Alternatively, it can be caused internally by a sensitivity to foods (cow's milk being the most common) or even inhalants such as house dust, cigarette smoke or pollens.

One gramme of vitamin C taken three times a day in the acute phase will be helpful but it is essential that this is accompanied by *plenty* of liquids.

DANDRUFF

There is a relationship between dandruff (dry, flakey particles of skin in the hair) and acne (spots on face, and sometimes on the upper part of the body). Acne is the blockage of the sebaceous (oil) glands whose purpose is to lubricate the skin and hair.

Selenium-containing shampoos such as Selsun and Lenium will help to control dandruff. They should be used with care, as toxicity can occur if instructions are not followed carefully. For this reason, I should recommend them to be used either intermittently with your usual shampoo, or alternatively for a limited period of time only.

Food allergies can be responsible for dandruff. Milk and milk products are a likely cause (just as they may cause cradle cap in babies). The most valuable supplement to relieve dandruff is zinc, which alone can help considerably. Oil of Evening Primrose, vitamin C, vitamin E, the B vitamins, especially B6 and cold pressed oils (sunflower or linseed) are all recommended. The cold pressed oils should be kept in tightly closed bottles in the fridge, to retain their valuable properties.

DEPRESSION

Depression is a condition of very low spirits which may or may not have an obvious cause. It is absolutely ghastly to suffer from depression and not much fun for those around you either. In fact, when one member of a family suffers from constant or recurrent depression, it can have a devastating effect on the others. It is one thing if he/she realizes his/her predicament and looks towards a remedy. It is quite another if the person does not, or will not, recognise his depression because any reference towards possible treatment will only antagonise.

I am referring here to clinical depression, and not to depression caused through circumstances such as bereavement, divorce or job loss. Devastating though these are, most people will, come to terms with such traumas.

There are hereditary tendencies which increase the likelihood of developing clinical depression. Having said that, it is also, to a certain extent, in the hands of chance as it may require a combination of several factors to converge together before someone sinks to a real 'low'.

If depression is prolonged or severe, it is regarded as an illness, and a severe clinical depression needs urgent medical attention, especially if there is even the remotest risk of suicide. About two per cent of the population is said to fall into this category annually, and women aged between twenty and fifty are the most likely to suffer. Their depression may last from a few days to several months. Some cases will get better even without treatment. Others will not. It is essential, therefore, to have a correct diagnosis. If depression is not due to circumstances, then it must be due to a chemical imbalance. This may be hormonal, examples of which are: following childbirth (when it requires urgent medical attention) or a hysterectomy; others include side-effects of the Pill or hormonal changes during the menopause. It is a common symptom in pre-menstrual syndrome (PMS) and migraine.

Depression is also common for a few days following a bout of 'flu or as the aftermath of shingles. In the case of the latter, vitamin B12 is often prescribed as a treatment, with a high success rate. It is also a common symptom of food or chemical allergies which are discussed in detail further on.

The symptoms associated with depression are a lack of interest in daily activities and therefore a poor performance at home and/or work, a loss of confidence, feelings of guilt, frequent crying or staring into space, loss of concentration, loss of memory, lack of interest in eating, disturbed sleep and/or wakefulness and wide mood swings varying from normal to suicidal. If there is a risk of suicide, then the sooner psychiatric help is sought the better.

Family and friends are much needed at such times to reassure the sufferer that he/she is cherished and needed and encourage him/her back into a normal life. This can be exhausting and time consuming and, although may seem to be getting nowhere, will pay dividends in the end.

Consult the doctor if the illness has lasted more than two weeks, if the patient cannot cope or is constantly hysterical or distressed, if the health of other members of the family is at risk and/or if suicide is considered a possibility.

The doctor will take a careful history of the patient and discuss problems and solutions. He will prescribe small quantities of drugs or maybe psychotherapy. If the depression is severe, he will refer the patient to a psychiatrist who will assess the situation and take over treatment. Again, this may be a drug treatment or psychotherapy or he may recommend a period of rest if he feels in-patient treatment would be beneficial. ECT, electro convulsive therapy, an electric current passed through the brain in carefully measured doses, is not so often used now due to the controversy surrounding it. However, in cases of severe depression, and some forms of schizophrenia, it has been life-saving when other treatments have failed.

It is important to remember that mental symptoms can also be due to an allergic reaction to a food or chemical inhalant. Either can be the sole cause or, alternatively, aggravating factors of other related or unrelated causes. Some of the mental symptoms most commonly found in food intolerance are depression and anxiety, often accompanied by excessive fatigue.

A very common cause of allergic depression is cow's milk. This is not a food intended for human beings, as Nature designed it for the young of its own species. How many times have you heard 'Milk is meant for calves'? However, we humans always know better and deprive the calves of what would be good for them in order to insist that we take what may be bad for us! Cow's milk has a different chemical composition and it contains a protein which is foreign to us. Also, most cows are given a maintenance dose of antibiotics, and sometimes they are treated with hormones as well, both of which pass through into the milk. If you can survive all this, then milk is a good source of calcium. Unfortunately a number of people cannot.

Other foods can be implicated in depression, and Dr Richard Mackarness (of *Not all in the Mind* fame) tells us of Dr Ted Randolph of Chicago who, as far back as 1958, used a fast of spring water for his patients who suffered from afflictions such as rheumatism, migraine, colitis, and depression with surprisingly good results.

Apart from milk, other most likely causes are wheat, corn, eggs, citrus fruits, cheese, sugar and artificial additives (especially colourings). Those which have been researched and found to be suspect are E102, E110, E120, E123, E127, E131, E132, E133, E142, E151, 154, E180, E210, E212, E220, E250, E251, E310–E312, E320, E321.

Caffeine, either in excess in the average person or even the minutest quantities in sensitive people, can cause depression. It is usually accompanied by other symptoms such as palpitations, shaking, nervousness and weight loss. Caffeine is to be found in some over-the-counter drugs as well as tea, coffee, chocolate and cola.

A number of allergic people are chemically sensitive, and may react to a wide range of things. Among the most likely are gas, paint, tobacco smoke and perfumes. A sensitivity to the latter can make life a nightmare as it is so impossible to avoid other people's perfumes when going into public places.

Another common cause of depression (and other allergic symptoms) is mould. Penicillin is made from mould (it is its ability to release a special toxin which kills the bacteria). Penicillin was the most brilliant discovery and is a commonly used and very effective antibiotic. Unfortunately, some people are allergic to it and may develop a wide range of allergic disorders – including rashes, breathing problems and depression.

We can produce psychiatric symptoms, including depression, if we become sensitive to our own *Candida*, a fungus which is in the natural flora in the gut of all human beings.

Depression may accompany asthma and hay fever either directly as a brain allergy, or indirectly, because both are such disabling conditions when suffered on a constant basis.

Depression is sometimes related to or aggravated by a trace mineral deficiency, possibly magnesium or zinc, a deficiency in vitamin C, B vitamins and folic acid; therefore, 1g of vitamin C daily and a strong preparation of B complex vitamins which contains folic acid and a good multi-mineral may well help. Exercising, say, half an hour a day for a minimum of four days a week will help combat depression and promote well-being.

The most important thing is to find the cause, whether this be allergy-related or not. Professional help can be invaluable in cases of severe depression. Only those who have suffered know how isolated you can feel but there *are* people you can turn to – professionals, and voluntary services such as the Samaritans, whose number you can find in your local directory. The latter operate a 24 hour telephone service and their doors are open from 10.00am to 10.00pm. There are Allergy Associations to help you discover the cause; these people *want* to help you – let them!

See also **Anxiety, Hypomania, Nervous Breakdown, Panic Attacks** and **Pre-menstrual Syndrome** (PMS).

DERMATITIS

Dermatitis means inflammation of the skin and is a generic term for all skin diseases. Contact dermatitis is caused by a sensitivity to things which come into contact with the outside of the body – such as soaps, detergents, washing powders, chemicals, airborne allergens, clothing, creams and cosmetics. An allergy to nickel is not uncommon. People with pierced ears who experience red, swollen ear lobes are usually reacting to the nickel with which the cheaper brands of earrings are made. Dermatitis can also be caused by an allergy to rubber (which may include rubber contraceptives). An allergy to rubber gloves is the one which usually comes to mind but what is less easily recognised is that footwear is often made of rubber too and this can cause swelling of the feet, cracked skin and other symptoms. Watch out for sponge rubber inner soles and elastic in the 'uppers'. Rubber wellington boots can be replaced by those made from PVC.

Substitutes for the above-mentioned allergens are: Simple Soap or other unperfumed soap, *Ecover* washing-up liquid and washing powder, or Boots' hypo-allergenic range, cotton clothing, hypo-allergenic, non-perfumed cosmetics, silver or rolled-silver earrings. A non-perfumed barrier cream will help to protect people with sensitive hands, and a hydrocortisone cream from your doctor is useful for emergencies – but do remember it is necessary to use this most sparingly.

A wide variety of skin sensitivities are not contact-related but are caused by reacting to common foods such as milk, wheat, eggs, coffee, yeast, citrus fruits, cheese, chocolate, artificial colourings, preservatives and other additives. Those particularly noted for causing skin complaints are E102, E131, E215–E219, E223, E321, 430 and 431.

Said to help to build up resistance to this type of reaction are vitamins A, B complex and E, and a good multi-mineral which includes zinc. Oil of Evening Primrose can work wonders with allergy-induced skin disorders.

See also **Acne, Eczema, Feet (swelling in)** and **Psoriasis**.

DEVELOPMENT IN CHILDREN, UNSATISFACTORY

There are very many different reasons for slow or unsatisfactory development in children but as this matter is of such prime importance to most of us, sometimes, through lack of experience, we worry unnecessarily. It is important to remember that there is a wide range of what is considered normal development. Children do things in their own time: one may put all his energies into running around and not be interested in learning to speak, another may be verbally fluent but sedentary, and so on.

Where a genetic defect or brain damage is diagnosed, much can be done – it is just a matter of finding the right people at the right time. Schools and other centres for the physically and mentally handicapped have some wonderfully dedicated members of staff whose experience can prove invaluable to your child and his rate of progress. It is important not to delay because the sooner he starts treatment the more effective it is likely to be. Your doctor will advise you who to contact.

If you are concerned that your child's mental or physical progress is not as it should be and all other causes have been eliminated, then it would be wise to consider the possibility of food or chemical allergy. Sometimes, I believe, there are some mis-diagnoses made of children who are suffering either physical or mental symptoms, including those considered backward or maladjusted. They may be no more nor less than undiagnosed hypersensitive individuals.

There are other children who suffer from colds, catarrh, sore throats, ear infections or chest complaints on a seemingly continuous basis whose symptoms are undoubtedly allergy-induced. The causes may be due to any so-called natural foods or natural or chemical inhalants, and there is positive evidence to prove that such problems have increased since such a wide range of artificial additives have become an accepted part of our western diet. Azo and coal-tar dyes and the benzoate preservatives must take a major share of the blame. All children suffering from allergies who are not already on one would improve on a good, healthy diet of fresh, natural foods. Their immune systems would benefit from a good boost of vitamins A and D and B complex and 1g of vitamin C daily. Younger children can take a multi-vitamin/mineral called *Junamac*, and *mini-Junamac* is suitable for babies after weaning.

I have only just scratched the surface of this vast and complex subject of allergy in children, mentioning only a few of the forms it may take. I suggest that you read as much as you can on the subject and try to find a paediatrician interested in allergy and environmental illness, or at least an experienced doctor. Contact an association – the names of those which have been established longest are at the back of this book. They have a wealth of experience behind them and will do all they can to help. Between you, you will win through!

See also **Allergy-induced Autism, Hyperactivity, Learning Difficulties and Behaviour Problems.**

DIARRHOEA

Diarrhoea is a very loose or liquid bowel movement. Sometimes people use the word 'diarrhoea' to indicate that stools have been passed several

D

times in one day. That in itself is not a symptom – it is the nature of the stools which is important. These should be well formed and passed without discomfort. People vary, and although we think of the 'average' as being once a day, there is no problem in going more or less frequently. A very loose stool, however, is an indication that something is wrong.

There are many different reasons for diarrhoea. In the acute form it is usually due to infection caused by food poisoning, in which case other members of the family may be at risk too. Much infection of this nature could be avoided if more people were conscious of the need for hygiene – not only those who prepare food but those who sit down and eat it too. Usually this type of infection will last only a few days. Occasionally there may be a more serious underlying cause, so if the symptoms are severe or persistent, or are accompanied by fever or abdominal pain, do consult your doctor. Consult him immediately if the patient is a baby or young child. They run a risk of becoming dehydrated. All their foods should be cut out and only a liquid diet of water or diluted fruit juices given. Lemon barley water is good and can be made from straining the water after boiling some barley, to which lemon and sugar or honey can be added. Plenty of liquid is very important for babies and small children to avoid any chance of their becoming dehydrated. This becomes even more vital if vomiting is present. Another useful drink is glucose water made with one pint of water to which a dessertspoonful of glucose and a pinch of salt have been added. No milk or milky drinks should be given. Patent medicines such as kaolin can be given to older children on a temporary basis, and *Dioralyte* and *Rehidrat* are good for diarrhoea too, but young children and babies must be given only those medicines prescribed especially for them.

Chronic diarrhoea where there is no apparent cause is nearly always allergic in origin. It is sometimes accompanied by migraine or other symptoms. By far the most common culprit is cow's milk followed by eggs and wheat, but any food can be responsible. Chemical allergies can cause diarrhoea, too, but unless the patient is known to be prone to chemical sensitivities, then foods are the more likely.

Another cause can be a digestive enzyme deficiency. The most common is a lack of the enzyme lactase required to metabolise the lactose. (milk sugar) in milk. This is known as lactose intolerance, and the diarrhoea will disappear as soon as milk is removed from the diet. The condition is inherited, and will be permanent, but once it is accepted and understood it will not present too much of a problem. There is a temporary form of lactose intolerance which occurs in both adults and children following a gastric infection; this is why milk must not be taken for several days afterwards.

For chronic diarrhoea sufferers, the following is recommended: vitamin A, B complex vitamins and acidophilus culture (two tablespoonfuls three times a day, or three capsules daily). Chronic sufferers may also benefit from taking extra iron.

See also **Abdominal Pain, Candidiasis, Colic, Coeliac Disease, Crohn's Disease Irritable Bowel Syndrome, Toddler Diarrhoea** and **Ulcerative Colitis.**

DIZZINESS

D

Dizziness is the feeling that someone has spun you round and round endlessly. It means that you have lost consciousness for a short time. There are many causes, including raised blood pressure, excess (or a sensitivity to) alcohol, excess (or a sensitivity to) caffeine, the effects of sleeping pills or other drugs, hot rooms or excessive fatigue. There are other more serious disorders such as Ménière's disease, middle ear problems and viral infections – also anaemia. Too much salt can cause abnormal fluid retention which can result in swollen legs and dizziness.

Dizziness can also be caused by various food allergies, the most common being coffee and other caffeine-containing foods or drinks. Suspect food additives are 621 (MSG), 622 and 623. Some people get this symptom through inhaling chemicals, such as car fumes, paint, cleaning materials etc.

People susceptible to dizzy spells may be short of manganese which is found in nuts, green leafy vegetables, peas, beets and egg yolks. It can also be bought as a supplement from health food shops.

See also **High Blood Pressure, Fainting Attacks** and **Ménière's Disease.**

DROWSINESS

Drowsiness can be caused by mental or physical fatigue. It is also a symptom of some medical conditions, one of the best known being myx-oedema (hypothyroidism). It is essential, therefore, to have a thorough medical check-up if you are feeling drowsy much of the time.

It can, of course, be an adverse reaction to certain drugs. Some antihistamines, especially, are known to cause people to feel dopey. (*Hismanal* and *Triludan* should not have this side-effect.) Poisoning is another reason for drowsiness, but other symptoms are likely to be present too.

Although not much is written about this subject with regard to allergy, this is a common allergic reaction to both foods and chemicals. (I know that if I had drunk a glass of milk prior to starting writing, I should now be yawning non-stop and finding it very hard to stay awake.)

Dextrose, which is made from corn, is a quick-acting sugar glucose; glucose tablets will also help to restore energy in normal circumstances. They have less effect in medical conditions, including allergic reactions, where the only real answer is to identify the cause.

See also **Zombie-like State.**

EARACHE AND ITCHY EARS

There are several causes of earache. A common one is a build-up of wax which can block the ear completely. The wax should be softened with olive oil for a few days before being syringed. People vary in the amount of wax they produce and, in general, the elderly are more prone to this. No one should try to remove hard wax themselves, or indeed put their finger in their ear for any reason as infection may be introduced in this manner.

Children are particularly susceptible to infections of the middle ear. When these follow on from a cold they are unavoidable and often require antibiotic treatment. However, recurrent infections which seem to appear out of the blue, when there has been little or no sign of a cold may, in fact, be due to food or inhalant allergens.

Perennial rhinitis can lead to the ear becoming blocked with mucus – this is called serous otitis or 'glue-ear' and is a common cause of deafness in children. It is essential to have this condition treated otherwise permanent damage can occur.

Allergy in the ears can cause itching, and when this becomes particularly pronounced it can be accompanied by weeping eczema which appears in the form of a colourless discharge. If you feel compelled to put your finger in your ear because the itching becomes unbearable, then do keep your fingernails short and your hands clean!

See also **Catarrah** and **Hay Fever**.

ECZEMA

Eczema is an inherited allergic susceptibility and is generally considered to be an affliction of childhood, although older children and adults can develop it too. Three-quarters of children affected show signs of it before they are a year old and, even if the causes are never found the majority will outgrow it sometime before adulthood.

Eczema consists of patches of red skin which erupt into blisters that often weep and then crust over. It is *very* itchy. In babies it can be on the head, the face, the arms, the legs or the nappy area. Not all nappy rashes are caused by eczema. They can be due to contact with ammonia, a chemical produced from urine by bacteria which normally live on moist skin. Zinc and castor oil cream will help to soothe the skin, whatever the cause. Leaving off nappies and exposing the bottom to the air will help too. However, it is important to have a medical diagnosis so you know what you are dealing with. Eczema on the head is called cradle cap and is usually caused by an allergy to cow's milk. Not surprisingly, babies suffering from eczema will be irritable, restless and they will cry a lot.

In older children, common places to find eczema are behind the ears, behind the knees, inside the elbows or on the wrists – in the moist areas of the body in fact, although any part of the body may be affected.

The most important fact to get over to parents, teachers or anyone in charge of a child with eczema is that the itching can be quite unbearable – a form of torture – far harder to bear than pain in many cases. If you have never experienced this, then consider yourself lucky and I ask you to take my word for it. It is my belief that to stop someone with eczema from scratching is a form of cruelty. Try to ensure that the child has clean hands and short fingernails in order to prevent infection entering the exposed skin, otherwise it could become painful and require antibiotic treatment. If you can persuade the child to rub rather than scratch this will help prevent breaking the skin. Even more important is to find a preparation which will keep the eczema at bay and help to relieve the itching. This will not necessarily be the first one your doctor prescribes. There are many creams and ointments made specifically for eczema but different ones suit different people. You will need to experiment. It is advisable to make it clear to teachers and other parents that the condition is not contagious in case they do not realise and are concerned about this.

It is useless expecting a child who suffers badly from eczema to concentrate on school work or anything else. The eczema dominates and will be made worse by stress. So if the child who cannot stop scratching irritates you, try not to show this but do what you can to help alleviate the itching. Expect the child to be more distressed at night as the warmth of his body in bed will aggravate the itching.

Obviously, whether for your child or yourself you will want a clear-cut diagnosis in order to start looking for a cause. (Even if your skin rash is diagnosed as positively *not* being eczema, this does not prohibit you looking for a cause.) All eczema needs treatment but it is essential to go to your doctor on any occasion when the eczema is accompanied by tenderness, boils or a discharge of pus. In chronic eczema the skin may become cracked and bleed. In some cases where the causes are not discovered, the condition can become life-long but, take heart, with all the knowledge you are gaining this will not apply to you!

Things you eat, breathe or touch, normally referred to as ingested, inhaled or contact allergens, can cause eczema. Eczema can also be caused by sensitivities to climate, wind, hot or cold temperatures or exercise, or it could be caused by a combination of any of these.

Food allergy is a major cause of eczema in children (and indeed adults too). The most common cause in babies is cow's milk – from which most formulas are made. It is now recognised (not before time) that 'breast is best', and the majority of mothers are able to breast-feed. (If you find that you are not producing breast-milk and all else fails, try excluding cow's milk yourself – you may be allergic to it without realising it.) Babies who are going to develop eczema are likely to do so within the first two months of their lives. If the milk feed is found to be the cause it can be changed to one of the soya-based formulas such as *Wysoy*, *Prosobee* and *Formula S* which are equally nutritious and

E

to which the necessary supplements have been added. Where there is a family history of allergy it may be advisable to avoid cow's milk in any form for the first year of the baby's life.

In a breast-fed baby who is very allergic to milk, the cow's milk from the mother's diet which passes through her breast-milk may be enough to cause eczema (or colic) in her baby. In a breast-fed baby who is less sensitive, but nevertheless allergic to cow's milk when taken in larger quantities, the symptoms will not show up until the baby is weaned and cow's milk is introduced direct.

Enough of babies. What about the rest of us? There is a controversy in the medical profession as to whether associated symptoms such as nevousness, irritability, fatigue and so on are part of the eczema syndrome or the result of the stress caused by the eczema. Ask a sufferer!! He will tell you that, as in any allergic reaction of any significance, you always get associated symptoms – *but* that being extremely itchy with only momentary relief is bound to make you nervous, irritable and exhausted, especially when those around you are fed up to the back teeth with your scratching. So the answer is – both are right.

Cow's milk is the most common cause of eczema in adults as well as children and babies but it is by no means the only one. Other known food allergens are wheat, other grains, eggs, citrus fruits, cheese, potatoes, fish, tomatoes, tea, coffee, chocolate, nuts, peanuts, beef and chicken. Even the fumes of such foods being cooked is enough to affect some highly sensitive people. One of the major causes over the last few decades has been artificial additives, especially azo dyes such as tartrazine and the benzoate preservatives. We must not forget that medicines can be the cause of eczema – in fact drugs can cause all manner of allergic reactions. When you learn that many medicines contain not one but several artificial colourings, this is not so surprising. Boots the Chemist has brought out a range of children's medicines free from artificial colourings. Let us hope that other manufacturers will have the sense to follow suit. Sometimes it is the antihistamines (the very drugs prescribed for allergies) which actually cause them! Aspirins, penicillin and hormone preparations can do the same.

I am grouping contactants and inhalants together because so often they are one and the same thing. Pollen, for example, can cause eczema in someone either because he breathes it in (where it will be absorbed into the blood stream) or because touching it will cause direct-contact eczema. The following are all possible allergens in this category: detergents and washing powders, household chemicals and cleaners, aerosol sprays, air fresheners, washing up liquid; wool, nylon and other synthetic fabrics, dyes in clothes, chemicals used in dry cleaning, surgical tape, hard water, chemicals used in gardening and at work; cosmetics, hairsprays, perfumes, deodorants, soaps, shampoos, powders, pharmaceutical creams and ointments – lanolin (wool fat) is a widely used additive in these; chemical dust, house dust, animal dander, newsprint, pollens, moulds, damp, indoor and outdoor pollution; house or garden plants, such as chrysanthemums and primulas, pollens and grasses, plastics, contraceptives, rubber (which is used for boots and shoes and from which elastic is made), and metals – mostly nickel (which is used for metal fastenings, cheap jewellery and watch straps). Quite a list, I think you will agree!

I now include some substitutes for those who happen to know what they are allergic to. For others they may be worth a try anyway.

In place of wool wear cotton, especially next to the skin as in underwear and nightwear. (See address of 'Cotton On' at back of book.) In place of rubber use PVC – gloves and wellington boots. Put cork inner soles in shoes.

If hard water is a problem, buy a water softener. Use soap powders or enzyme-free detergents. *Ecover* is tolerated by most people. The same company also does a biodegradable washing up liquid. Boots the Chemist does a whole range of hypo-allergenic household materials. In place of soap use an emulsifying ointment such as Wash E45. In place of hand cream use Cream E45. Bath oils help dry skin. Avoid highly perfumed ones. Baby oil is good – as is Bath E45. These are usually well tolerated. Use hypo-allergenic cosmetics. These are perfume-free. There are various makes around, but Boots' own make is probably the most reasonably priced. Use an unperfumed moisturiser at night. Micropore tape is well tolerated by those who cannot use elastoplast.

If nickel is a problem avoid cheap jewellery. One of the most common problem areas is pierced ears. Silver or rolled silver, or steel prongs, are usually safe. Replace woollen blankets, feather pillows and duvets with cotton blankets and/or polyester duvets and pillows. Keep carpets and mattresses well hoovered. Never use a horse-hair mattress. Keep curtains and furniture dust-free.

Eczema can appear within minutes of contact with the allergen, whether it be ingested or inhaled, or through bodily contact, or the reaction may be delayed for several hours. Some people who are less severely afflicted will only react to large amounts of an offending substance and therefore it may take a build-up of several days before the eczema appears. Whilst it is vital to look for the causes (and a cause there certainly is) it is also very important not to deny the relief that medication can bring to the unfortunate sufferer. There are a number of creams and ointments made for eczema. Corticosteroids, of which the most common is hydrocortisone, are the most commonly prescribed and, providing they are used sparingly, will be effective without being harmful. In extreme cases antihistamines can be prescribed to control the itching. Some antihistamines cause drowsiness which will add to the patient's problems unless used at night when they will be helpful! *Triludan* and *Hismanal* should not have this effect. Cases where the eczema has become infected may require antibiotic treatment. One of the safest and best aids to control eczema is to take Oil of Evening Primrose. This can be prescribed by your doctor but is also available in health food shops.

E

As eczema patients are considered by some authorities to be deficient in essential fatty acids it can be well understood why this should be so effective. Other sources of essential fatty acids are wheatgerm oil, linseed oil, sunflower oil, safflower oil, soybean oil, peanuts, sunflower seeds, walnuts, pecans, almonds and avocados.

A dry, eczematous skin can be caused by a vitamin and mineral deficiency. Good supplements to take are vitamins A and E, B complex vitamins, multi-minerals, plus extra zinc and acidophilus culture.

The great thing is to experiment and find out what works best for you.

ENURESIS (BED-WETTING)

Enuresis means bed-wetting. Children vary enormously at what age they gain control of their bladders. At first they will become dry during the day and nappies can be discarded. For a time they will need to wear them at night and can be 'pottied' before the parents retire to bed themselves.

Everyone has their own system. Too rigid an attempt to potty train a child may have the reverse effect. A child will show when he is ready to take responsibility, and when he does so is the time to take advantage of this, even if it means taking a potty wherever you go!

Some children will have stopped wetting themselves early on while others may not succeed until the age of four or five, and some will take longer. If children drink a lot this may add to the problem. Whilst you do not wish to restrict their fluids it may be helpful to withdraw the bedtime drink. Sometimes a bed-wetting child is simply a heavy sleeper and fails to wake up. You may need to wake him yourself. Even if this goes on for some time, it is less of an ordeal than changing a bed and lets him retain his self-esteem.

If your child is constantly wetting the bed, or if you are worried about him, ask your doctor to do a urine check in case he is suffering from an infection.

Diabetes, though less likely, is another possible cause. Usually there is no problem – the child is just taking a little longer to learn control. Sometimes distress or emotional trauma is the root cause and, occasionally, bed-wetting can start again after being dry if the child has been upset. Refraining from criticising a child who has had an accident and praising him when he has remained dry will go a long way to help overcome the problem when the cause is emotional. No one wants to be a bed-wetter, and whatever the reason it is not intentional.

A few people will go on to being bed-wetting teenagers and even adults but, once understood, this problem is not too difficult to overcome. There are two aspects to it – one is control over the bladder and the other is how often the bladder needs to be emptied. If it is much more often than usual, this is known as 'frequency', and adults have the problem as much as children. When it is accompanied by a burning sensation, it is known as 'cystitis'.

Infection must be ruled out first, but the principal cause is food allergy which can cause a very frequent need to urinate. Antihistamines may give temporary relief (and can be used to prove the point) but it is essential to discover the cause. The most common cause is cow's milk, followed by wheat, citrus fruits, eggs, chocolate, tomatoes, cola, nuts and food additives, especially colourings. Orange squash is often found to be the culprit. Inhalant allergens are sometimes to blame, and these include pollen, house dust, mould and cigarette smoke. The individual must be given every opportunity to discover the cause of this distressing and embarrassing symptom.

See also **Cystitis**. (Urinary incontinence in the elderly and disabled is a separate issue not covered in this book.)

EPILEPSY

Epilepsy is a form of seizure (fit). Seizures are caused by abnormal electrical activity in the brain. As this spreads through the brain it causes a convulsion. The two best known forms of epilepsy are *grand mal* and *petit mal*. In *grand mal* the patient loses consciousness, stiffens, and his limbs begin to twitch. He may go blue, froth at the mouth and bite his tongue. He will remain unconscious for some minutes after the attack and this may be followed by a feeling of tiredness and confusion.

At the start of an epileptic fit lay the patient on his side with plenty of space around him; loosen his collar and do not try to restrict his movements. If possible push a clean, rolled up hanky or a metal spoon between his teeth to prevent him biting his tongue. When he returns to consciousness, try to curb your own fears and reassure the patient. A doctor should always be called for an epileptic fit if it is unexpected or prolonged.

In *petit mal*, which usually occurs in pre-adolescent children, the child will lose consciousness for a few seconds only and look quite blank before carrying on with what he was doing. He will probably be unaware that anything has happened.

Fits can be caused by injury at birth, certain serious illnesses, the effects of drugs or drink, a stroke or a head injury. In certain susceptible people the causes can be environmental and can be triggered by stress, bright or flashing lights or even watching television. Going without food for too long can provoke an attack, as can too little sleep.

Certain foods and drinks can cause fits, the most common ones being alcohol, coffee, tea, sugar, chocolate, wheat, milk and milk products, cheese, citrus fruits and artificial additives, especially colourings. The sweetener, aspartame (also known as *Canderel* or *Nutrasweet*) in high doses has been known to trigger epilepsy. Epileptic seizures can also be caused by chemical inhalants. Obviously, in some circumstances the cause can be a combination of any of these factors.

If you wish to investigate the dietary approach by going onto an

E

elimination diet, it would be better to try to find an experienced clinical ecology doctor to supervise you. Unmasking food allergens and reintroducing them later can cause a more severe reaction, and you have to be prepared for this.

Taurine, a non-essential amino acid in combination with glutamic and aspartic acids is said to be helpful for seizures, but the best thing would be to discuss this with a nutritionally orientated doctor. There may be vitamin or mineral deficiencies, so a strong multi-vitamin/mineral supplement would not come amiss.

One of the most distressing aspects of being an epileptic is other people's attitudes. Therefore I suggest that you explain to, and reassure, them if you suffer in this way and they, in turn, knowing what to expect, will stop feeling frightened and will be able to help and reassure you.

See also **Convulsions, Hypoglycaemia.**

EYE CONDITIONS

There are many serious disorders which cause eye symptoms, and a doctor should always be consulted even if only to eliminate these. Inflammation of the eyes is very often caused by a germ and this will need medical treatment.

One of the most common problems of the eyes is when a foreign body enters, and if it cannot be easily removed this will require a visit to the eye hospital or casualty department of your local hospital. Chemicals inadvertently splashed into the eyes can be dangerous and require urgent medical treatment. Keep pouring water into them until the doctor arrives.

Eye problems are a common cause of headaches. This may simply mean that you need a pair of glasses or (if you already have some) that the lenses need to be changed. Most people over the age of fifty require glasses. Some people suffer from eye problems as a result of sensitivity to light and they may require dark glasses with polarised lenses.

When no other cause can be found, allergy should be considered. Typical allergy symptoms of the eye are:

Puffiness under eyes
Dark circles under eyes (known as allergic shiners)
Swollen eyelids (which may be red and itchy)
Dry eyes
Watery eyes
Sensitive eyes
Recurrent styes
Red, itchy, watery eyes as a symptom of hay fever
Red, sore or itchy eyes as a symptom of conjunctivitis (this can also be
    caused by infection)

Blurred vision when it is associated with eating certain foods or coming into contact with certain inhalants.

Causes of eye allergies can be just about any foods or airborne allergens such as pollens, smoke, fumes or any other chemicals. Some people even suffer from an adverse reaction to the preservatives used in the cleaning fluids for contact lenses. Certain over-the-counter eye washes can cause allergic reactions, occasionally making the eyeball swell alarmingly. Eye cosmetics can cause problems but there are several brands of hypo-allergenic ones around which should be safe for most people.

Opticrom is a good anti-allergy eye preparation but this has to be prescribed by your doctor. It is better to use only those preparations prescribed by your doctor or recommended by your chemist.

Vitamin A has wonderful properties for restoring eyes to a healthy state, whatever the problem. It can help to counteract night blindness and weak eyesight and aid in the treatment of many eye disorders. It helps to cure styes, bloodshot eyes and a burning sensation of the eyes. The average adult dose is 10,000ius daily; however, under no circumstances exceed the stated dose. Vitamin B2 is also of value but (unless prescribed by someone trained in nutritional medicine) it is better taken in the form of a preparation of B complex vitamins, where all the B vitamins are balanced.

See also **Conjunctivitis, Hay Fever,** and **Vision, Disturbance of.**

E

F

FAINTING ATTACKS

Fainting is a temporary loss of consciousness and collapse. Although the patient turns very pale, most faints are not serious and last only a few minutes. The causes are either emotional – fear, the sight of blood, bad news, shock, etc, or physical – heat, fever, pregnancy, prolonged standing, injury, hunger, etc. People suffering from low blood sugar (multiple allergy sufferers and diabetics for example) will feel faint after a few hours without food, and this can be relieved by taking a glucose tablet, an apple or a warm drink. Occasionally, fainting can be a symptom of heart disease or anaemia and, if, in doubt, see your doctor. He should be consulted anyway if there are other symptoms present or if the fainting fits continue.

If you feel faint, sit down and put your head between your legs until the feeling passes. Another means of preventing fainting is to keep wriggling your toes. This helps your blood supply return to your heart from your legs. If you see someone about to faint, catch him if you can, lay him flat, loosen his collar and wait for the faint to pass.

People who repeatedly feel faint for no good reason might well find that it is caused by the effects of caffeine, which is a drug and potentially toxic. Even the smallest amounts can affect some people. Other foods, such as eggs and milk, etc can be responsible, of course, as can be artificial additives, but coffee is the most common. Inhalant allergens such as gas, car fumes, perfumes, aerosol sprays or other inhaled chemicals can cause fainting.

See also **Dizziness, Hypoglycaemia.**

FATIGUE

Fatigue, known also as apathy, lethargy, listlessness, exhaustion, weariness and excessive tiredness can be caused by a hangover, fever, infection, emotional trauma, anxiety and insomnia. It is also a symptom of illnesses such as anaemia, myxoedema and other serious disorders, so it should always be checked if in doubt. Bereavement can cause a feeling of great exhaustion from which it may take weeks or months to recover.

Fatigue can be a symptom of allergy. It is often accompanied by tension when it becomes known as the tension/fatigue syndrome and will probably be linked to muscle weakness as well. It is a common symptom of angioedema, migraine and irritable bowel syndrome, all well documented allergic disorders.

Extreme exhaustion is also a symptom of post-viral syndrome, which lowers the immune system causing susceptibility to allergies. This type of excessive tiredness is not helped by rest, and sufferers are constantly below par, may be nervous, anxious, unable to concentrate, have headaches, sleep badly and have dark circles under their eyes.

Causes may be environmental or seasonal changes. (Hence the reason why asthma and hay fever sufferers are victims too.) Other causes are allergies to foods, drugs or inhalants. The most common cause, however, is coffee, as the caffeine in it acts directly upon the nervous system. Even the most minute amounts can affect some people. It produces an almost immediate sense of clearer thought and lessens fatigue – until the effects wear off, when it is likely to produce the opposite effect. It is believed by the medical profession in general that those people who are heavy coffee drinkers (five cups a day or more) have a greater chance of developing other diseases, including heart disease and some forms of cancer. Pregnant women are better off without it. Tea, chocolate and cola also contain caffeine, so it is as well to keep a check on these too. Other foods, such as cow's milk, wheat and eggs can cause fatigue too, as can drugs and chemical inhalants.

Many supplements are said to be helpful in combating fatigue. These are folic acid and pantothenic acid (B vitamins), vitamin E, biotin, iron and manganese (mineral supplements), certain amino acids, and ginseng. Iron should be taken by anyone who has suffered a severe blood loss. Vegetarians and menstruating women are particularly prone to anaemia and can help prevent this by taking an iron supplement.

See also **Myalgic Encephalomyelitis** (ME) and **Tension/Fatigue Syndrome**.

FEET, SWELLING IN

Swollen feet (also legs and ankles) may be associated with heart or kidney disease so, if in any doubt, consult your doctor.

Swelling of ankles (and feet) after middle age is not uncommon and does not necessarily indicate serious illness. During pregnancy some women develop swollen ankles and feet. Other causes for swollen feet include obesity, hot weather, prolonged standing, arthritis, gout and a sprain or fracture. If swelling persists, consult your doctor.

If none of the above apply it is possible that you are suffering from an allergy to a substance used in the manufacture of your footwear, irrespective of whether or not you are wearing socks, stockings, or neither. The swelling may affect one or both feet and could even extend to ankle and leg. Other forms of allergy, such as eczema, may be present also.

The most common allergy is to the chemicals used in curing rubber. If this is the case, you will need to avoid shoes which have elastic inserts or rubber inner soles. (These can be replaced by cork soles.) Those people who suffer from a more severe allergy will need to avoid shoes which contain any rubber at all, including even the soles. Wellington boots are usually made from rubber, so replace those with boots made from PVC. They look the same and are no more expensive.

Apart from rubber chemicals, the most likely allergen is found in some adhesives and is, namely, *para-tertiary butyl phenol formaldehyde*. A relatively small number of people suffer from an allergy to the tanning substance in leather. Clarks and other shoe manufacturers can provide lists of shoes which do not contain these substances.

For further information please send £1.00 to the British Footwear Manuacturers' Federation, Royalty House, 72 Dean Street, London W1V 5HB for their booklet *Footwear for Special Needs*.

FEVER (RAISED TEMPERATURE)

F

A fever is not a specific illness – it is symptomatic of illness being present and is the body's means of fighting back. Babies and children are the most likely to produce very high temperatures, adults less so, and the elderly may even be without a fever in spite of serious illness being present if their bodily resources are unable to fight back. The average normal temperature is 37° Centigrade or 98.4° Fahrenheit, although there are people whose normal temperature is one degree above or one degree below this.

If you have a baby with a fever, whatever his temperature, you should call your doctor. If you have a child with a temperature of 102° or over, call your doctor. If your child has a lower temperature but looks ill, is flushed, is not eating, has a pain or is vomiting, or you are concerned, call your doctor.

If fever persists in an adult for more than a day or two, or if there are other serious symptoms present, or if the patient is shaking or shivering severely or cannot stop his teeth chattering, seek medical advice straight away.

Some children run high temperatures, with other symptoms present, on a recurring basis for no apparent reason. If all other possible causes have been eliminated, a food or chemical allergy could be the cause. Investigations have been done showing that children who were challenged with certain foods developed fevers; these could be quite sudden and were sometimes high. The same thing can happen with adults, although this is relatively rare.

Fever robs the body of its most essential nutrients, and the longer or more serious the illness the more depleted the body will be. The infectious diseases of childhood, for example, will leave a child particularly low in nutrients.

Recommended are a good multi-mineral, a good multi-vitamin plus 1g a day of vitamin C. This is suitable for children as well as adults and will be beneficial both during a fever and in the convalescent period which follows.

'FLU-LIKE SYMPTOMS

Different types of viruses will cause different kinds of 'flu but most of them will include symptoms such as fever, shivering, feeling ill, cold, sore throat, cough, catarrh and aching all over. The fever and other symptoms will probably have abated in less than a week but the cough and catarrh may continue for some time. Depression is common for a few days following 'flu. When 'flu is accompanied by sickness we usually refer to it as gastric 'flu.

There is no effective treatment other than bed rest, keeping warm, taking plenty of fluids and pain-killers such as aspirins (if they can be tolerated) or paracetemol. Antibiotics are of use only in secondary infections such as bronchitis or tonsilitis. Vaccines (given in October) are advisable for anyone at risk, such as the elderly, but they will not protect against all viruses.

Viral infections lower the body's defences and make us more susceptible to allergic reactions than we would otherwise be. In this hyper-sensitive state any allergic reactions will be more severe so it is essential that after a dose of 'flu we build up our immune systems with the necessary supplements. This will help rally our defences to kill off any lurking bugs, thereby preventing the development of post-viral syndrome.

It is important to realise that the reverse can happen also and that it is possible to have allergic reactions which mimic 'flu. This can be difficult to recognise and it may be only after someone has 'flu several times in fairly rapid succession that suspicion is aroused. If the patient is a known allergy sufferer, this makes the chances more likely. The causes may be inhaled fumes or other chemicals or any foods. Food additives, wheat, citrus fruits, milk, pork, strawberries and alcohol have all been incriminated.

Supplements which should be taken for a minimum of two to three weeks following 'flu are vitamin A, vitamin E, 1g of vitamin C daily and acidophilus culture. It is advisable also to keep up your intake of extra fluids.

F

GENERAL FEELING OF BEING UNWELL

Many people who suffer from allergies can feel unwell in such a general way (possibly with no other symptoms) that they have difficulty in finding the words to express exactly how they feel. They are in no doubt, however, that they *do* feel ill. This has been described to me in many different ways, often hesitatingly, but the phrase I think most explicit is 'all-over-grottiness'.

All I can say is that if your doctor has excluded anaemia or any other reason why you should feel under par, then it could be due to something you are eating, drinking or inhaling. If you are a known allergy sufferer already then this is all the more likely.

If you improve on a change of diet or environment, or this feeling is connected to any particular season, then consider the odds overwhelming. Other reasons could be lack of essential nutrients, exercise, fresh air, or sleep, or excessive worry. Discover which by a process of elimination.

GINGIVITIS

Gingivitis is inflammation of the gums which become bright pink and bleed on brushing. It can start in childhood or, indeed, at any other time. If left untreated, gingivitis can lead to irreversible damage and loss of teeth. Its cause has been attributed to an allergy to certain foods by some people, although the general belief is that it is due to lack of oral hygiene. However, this is not always the case, and another cause has been found to be an acute lack of vitamin C. Taking 3g of vitamin C daily (and reducing to 1g following an improvement) will in many cases cause the condition to clear up completely.

GLANDS, SWOLLEN

When we use the term 'swollen glands', we are usually referring to the lymphatic or lymph glands, the major ones of which are situated in the neck, armpits and the groin. They filter out the toxins which accumulate when a germ enters the body, thus causing the glands to swell.

Whilst infection is the most common cause, the immune system can be affected adversely by an allergy, and can cause lymph nodes to swell even though no germ is present. Foods, food additives and inhalants can all be responsible. The most commonly incriminated foods are milk, wheat, pork, citrus fruits and alcohol. Vitamin C is most beneficial whatever the cause. It has excellent anti-infection properties and is also a natural antihistamine. One gram taken three times a day whilst the glands are still swollen, followed by 1g daily after that, is the recommended dose.

GOUT

Gout is a form of painful arthritis caused by crystals of uric acid forming in the joints. The most common joint to be affected is that in the big toe. There is usually a sudden onset of acute pain and the patient feels ill. Once started it is likely to continue, and repeated attacks can lead to chronic arthritis. It affects adult men, rarely women. It can be controlled with treatment, including anti-inflammatory medicines, and is likely to improve with age!

Gout is generally believed to be triggered by certain foods, particularly the more starchy or sugary ones, including alcohol and beer in particular. It is believed to develop when someone takes more starchy or sugary foods than the body can cope with. The drug allopurinol reduces the level of uric acid in the body, thereby preventing recurrences. The best natural cure is yeast, which is an excellent source of protein and natural B complex vitamins and helps to reverse gout. Avoid flavour enhancers 631 and 635 and Inosine 5.

G

HALITOSIS (BAD BREATH)

Halitosis can be due to poor care of teeth and gums. Regular, careful, daily brushing should dispense with any problems in this direction. More complex dental matters can be dealt with by your dentist.

Halitosis is also caused by throat and other infections. Very occasionally it can be due to more serious disorders but then it is likely that other symptoms would be present.

Bad breath can also be due to the result of eating things such as garlic, onions and spicy foods. This is usually fairly easily recognised and no doubt someone will inform you pretty smartly.

Halitosis can also be caused by an allergic reaction to a food – the most common being milk, wheat and artificial additives. Anyone can be affected from infancy to old age. Babies with bad breath often suffer from colic too, which is another indication that this is due to a food sensitivity – probably milk in their case.

People, especially the young, sometimes worry unnecessarily that they have bad breath. You can test yourself by cupping your hands over your nose and mouth as you breathe out. If your breath smells alright to you, then the chances are it does to other people too. It is my experience that those people who really do suffer from halitosis seldom worry about it. They usually insist upon coming up really close and talking for a very long time.

Mouth washes can help – on a temporary basis – but people prone to allergies to food additives may be sensitive to the colourings in them as, indeed, they may be to coloured toothpastes. Perhaps the most useful aid to bad breath is chlorophyll – a natural product, and therefore Nature's deodorant. It can be taken in either tablet or liquid form.

B vitamins, amino acids, acidophilus culture and zinc are all said to help counteract the problem of halitosis.

HALLUCINATIONS

A hallucination is the belief that something which does not exist has been seen, felt or heard. If this is a minor event, and the person concerned realises it was a trick of the imagination, then this is of no significance.

However, if someone has seen rabbits dancing on the wallpaper or had a conversation with Napoleon then this suggests a serious brain disorder. The question is – what has caused it? A high temperature and delirium might be one reason, delirium tremens (DTs) another. The latter is a serious condition usually found in habitual drinkers. Hallucinations can also be caused by street drugs such as LSD or medical drugs such as Levodopa. They can also be induced by hypnosis. The medical profession will investigate if any physical abnormality is suspected.

Sometimes in schizophrenia the patient will hallucinate. Some forms

H

of schizophrenia are caused (or aggravated) by food intolerances and, if these were detected and eliminated, the condition could be stabilised. The trouble is that the majority of schizophrenics will never be given the opportunity to check these out. As Dr Richard Mackarness says in his book *Chemical Victims*: 'Chemical changes in the body brought about by something one has eaten can affect the central nervous system and alter the consciousness enough to produce hallucinations or imaginary fears.' I can find no documentation on the foods which most commonly cause hallucinations, therefore I simply suggest as the most likely suspects coffee, tea, cola and chocolate (because they contain caffeine), sugar (because it is known to cause personality changes), cheese (because it is said to 'play tricks on the brain'), and wheat and milk (because they are the most common of all food allergens). Food additives are always suspect, especially the azo and coal-tar dyes.

To summarise, causes can be a high fever, alcohol abuse, contact with concentrated toxins or an adverse reaction to drugs, foods or pollutants. Another reason, not yet mentioned, can be a severe deficiency in trace minerals which are very necessary for the proper functioning of our bodies. It has recently been discovered, for example, that schizophrenics are zinc deficient.

Anyone who 'hears voices' or sees things which, for the rest of us, do not exist, may be very low on zinc, and I suggest extra zinc and a good multi-mineral/multi-vitamin supplement.

HAY FEVER

Hay fever is inflammation of the lining of the nose which then becomes blocked and feels stuffy. Excess mucus is produced; this runs from the nose and can drip into the throat, causing soreness and/or itching and coughing. Although it is not always easy to differentiate initially between hay fever and a cold, if the roof of your mouth and your ears *continue* to itch this is more likely to denote allergy.

The symptoms of hay fever are unpleasant and varied. Some people may suffer from one symptom only and others from several. These are catarrh, runny nose, blocked nose, frequent sneezing, sore and watery eyes, sore throat, and cough. Further complications can be blocked ears and nasal polyps (small tumour-like growths in the nose which can be operated on if necessary). When people suffer to any degree, this dulls the brain, and sinusitis and/or headaches can add to the problem. Undoubtedly the patient will feel tired and irritable. Emotional upsets exacerbate the condition. Consult your doctor if you need help, if the hay fever gets too severe, if deafness develops, or if you have a headache not relieved by medication. He will prescribe the necessary treatment, possibly arrange for an allergy test and check for nasal polyps.

Apart from the well-documented grass-pollen hay fever, many other substances can cause hay fever symptoms. Among these are flower and

H

tree pollens, grass and weed pollens (recognised in USA), dust, house-dust mites, household chemicals, animal dander, moulds, atmospheric changes, pollution, cosmetics, perfumes, tobacco fumes, feathers, foods, drinks, food additives and medications. Some nose drops contain drugs which help at first but aggravate the condition in the long term. Some antihistamines have side-effects and bring on the very symptoms they are supposed to cure.

The following is advice to hay fever sufferers in the grass pollen season. It is equally suitable for sufferers of any other unavoidable seasonal allergy.

1. Start taking antihistamine tablets from 1 June. *Hismanal* or *Triludan*, which can be prescribed or bought over the counter without pre-scription, have been found to be highly effective for most people and do not cause drowsiness or other side-effects. Some people swear by homeopathic treatments so obviously these are effective too provided that the instructions are carefully followed and they are *not* taken at the same time as eating or drinking.
2. Take 1g of vitamin C daily. Vitamin C is a natural antihistamine. In fact, in severe cases of hay fever, up to 3g a day (taken in three separate doses) can be taken for a limited period. Buy this in its pure form as either Boots' vitamin C powder or one of the Cantassium products sold in many health food shops. Never choose the fizzy, soluble tablets as they contain artificial additives. In cases where people feel very run-down, I suggest supplementing this with a good artificial additive-free preparation of B complex vitamins and a multi-mineral.
3. Ask your doctor if he/she would prescribe *Rynacrom* nasal spray and/or *Opticrom* eye drops. These are forms of sodium cromoglycate which is known for its safety record and lack of side-effects.
4. Avoid grass and all other known allergens as these will lower your allergy-tolerance level and make your hay fever worse.
5. Get more than average rest – you need it. The stress of constant hay fever is using up your energy resources.
6. Buy an ioniser. The best known is 'Mountain Breeze' which can be obtained from Boots the Chemist and some health food shops. They used to cost £40.00. The price is coming down as these are becoming more popular. Ionisers produce the valuable negative ions which are good for you and displace the stale positive ones which are not. Car ionisers are available too.

By following these simple instructions you should find that your symptoms are under control and may even disappear altogether. I suggest following these precautions until mid-July.

Another possibility for grass pollen allergy sufferers (or indeed if you suffer from any of the 'accepted' allergies) is to be desensitised under the

H

NHS. This is a more complicated procedure than it used to be; it involves a series of visits to a hospital and a two-hour wait following the injection to ascertain whether there will be an adverse reaction. Inevitably, facilities are more limited than when this treatment was available in surgery. To add to the problem there are now more sufferers than previously because of increased pollutants. Atmospheric toxins combine with pollens, moulds and so on to push people over their tolerance threshold.

I recommend using a medical mask (obtainable from chemists' shops) for house dust/house-dust mite allergy sufferers when doing your house-work. Other useful tips are that a damp cloth is preferable to a duster and hoovering is preferable to brushing. Vacuum your bedroom daily and your mattress also (unless you prefer to use a plastic cover). Give your bed clothes a good airing as often as you can because sunshine and dry air are good for getting rid of dust mites.

For people who suffer from chronic or spasmodic hay fever which is not seasonal, and for which they have not yet discovered the cause, alternative possibilities exist. Many people use a wide range of perfumed items on their bodies and in their homes without ever realising that, unless otherwise stated, these are made from chemicals. They include perfumed toiletries, soaps, air fresheners, cleaning materials and so on. These should be removed from use to see if the symptoms clear before embarking upon an elimination diet (see Chapter 5).

Among the foods and drinks which can cause these symptoms are milk, wheat, eggs, chocolate, peas, beans, tomatoes, onions, potatoes, beef, citrus fruits, fish and coffee. Odours from foods can also cause hay fever in very sensitive people. Both alcoholic and non-alcoholic drinks can cause hay fever and/or wheezing too. In the alcoholic drinks it is very often the sulphur dioxide which is reponsible, and in the non-alcoholic fizzy drinks one or more of a wide range of chemical additives. The colourings E102 and E142 have been implicated in hay fever.

In June 1989, the *Daily Telegraph* quoted Oxford researchers who stated that wheezing illnesses such as hay fever and asthma were caused by the presence of a single rogue gene. The research study published in the *Lancet* was carried out by Dr Julian Hopkin, consultant physician at the Churchill Hospital, and Dr William Cookson, research fellow at the John Radcliffe Hospital. The *Daily Telegraph* states: 'Although they are not yet able to identify the gene they have narrowed down the area of search and say new methods of prevention are on the horizon.'

So until such a time, and whatever the cause of your hay fever, whether it is chronic, spasmodic or seasonal, there is much you can do to help yourself. Try to discover and eliminate the causes first and foremost, and then build up your resistance with supplements. I recommend up to 3g of vitamin C daily, a good multi-mineral and a strong preparation of B complex vitamins. There is always an answer – it is just a case of finding it.

See also **Catarrh** and **Sinusitis**.

H

HEADACHES

Children as well as adults can suffer from headaches. They are sometimes accompanied by a feeling of disorientation or confusion. The causes are wide ranging and may be psychological or physical. Some of the common ones are prolonged concentration (such as during a long spell of driving), overwork, anxiety or worry, mental fatigue, tension, rising blood pressure, travelling, side-effects of drugs, eye-strain, hunger, smoking, lack of sleep, hangover or an injury such as a bump on the head. Headaches can be a symptom of migraine or sinusitis or a symptom of an infection, when they may or may not be accompanied by fever. Serious disorders such as brain tumours are much less likely but need to be eliminated. Headaches which come on in the evening, when the patient is tired, may be tension headaches.

Sometimes people do not realise that their eyes need testing or their lenses changing, and eye-strain can be a cause of headaches. Plain, simple overdoing things (which cannot always be avoided) is another possibility – as is emotional stress when the patient may have difficulty in coming to terms with the situation. In this case there is a need to discuss the problems with your doctor who may be able to refer you for some sort of therapy. He can also prescribe pain-killers but, hopefully, other non-drug forms of relief can be found so that these will be needed only short-term or in an emergency.

Consult your doctor when a headache follows an injury (especially if the patient is drowsy) and if other symptoms are present such as vomiting, visual distortion, stiffness of the neck or back. Consult him also if your headache has persisted for more than three days and/or if it fails to respond to pain-killers. Headaches are one of the symptoms of migraine in adults and the main symptom of migraine in children. Relaxation and rest in a darkened room is the best home treatment, taking pain-killers such as paracetemol or aspirin (if they can be tolerated) every four hours.

Recurrent headaches which cannot be explained by the medical profession when all other possibilities (including serious disorders) have been discounted are likely to be due to food intolerance or chemical sensitivity. These reactions may be rapid or delayed. Among the most likely foods are coffee, tea, chocolate, cola, milk, nuts, wheat, corn, cheese, fish, eggs, citrus fruits and tomatoes. The following food additives have been implicated in headaches – E102, E281, E282, 621, 622 and 623.

Chemical sensitivities may be due to gas or oil in the home, cigarette smoke, car exhaust fumes and other pollutants. Allergies to pollens, moulds, straw and hay etc are all possibilities – as are adverse reactions to perfumes and household chemicals. Headaches are also a common symptom of *withdrawal* from caffeine (and other foods), as may be experienced in an elimination diet. If a bad headache is anticipated, it can be lessened by giving up the suspect food on a gradual basis –

the choice is up to the individual. Withdrawal from steroids and other drugs which have been taken over a prolonged period may also provoke a headache. All women should be told (but of course they never are) that the contraceptive pill is a steroid and can cause a variety of symptoms including headaches and, indeed, full-blown migraines also.

Fresh air, exercise and regular meals will help you to combat headaches, and relaxation and yoga are good too. Relaxed people are less likely to suffer from headaches. (However, it is fair to say that only people who do not suffer from headaches are likely to be relaxed!) Where allergies are concerned, there is no doubt that any stress will aggravate an allergic reaction, so freedom from stress must lessen it.

I recommend a good preparation of B complex vitamins, 1g of vitamin C daily, a multi-mineral supplement and dolomite (a combination of magnesium and calcium). These will go a long way towards building up your immune system. Try to discover the cause of the headaches. If you write down where you have been, what you have done, what you have eaten and drunk in the twenty four hours prior to starting your headache, and compare notes after two or three times, you should come up with a common factor. If there is more than one cause you may need to go on to an elimination diet.

See also **Migraine** and **Sinusitis**.

HEART CONDITIONS

Some congenital defects of the heart are caused by the mother contracting an illness such as German measles when pregnant. This is why we now have a German measles (Rubella) vaccine given to girls before puberty. A baby's heart can also be damaged by certain drugs – even self-prescribed ones – so it is essential to discuss this matter with your doctor in the very early stages of pregnancy.

As for the rest of us, to give ourselves the very best chance of avoiding any form of heart disease we need to eat a good, healthy diet of fresh (not processed) foods, be non-smokers, cut down on sugar, salt and alcohol consumption, try to maintain the ideal weight for our age and sex and take regular, moderate exercise. Swimming and walking are said to be good in this respect. We are recommended to avoid saturated (animal) fats because they contribute to higher levels of cholesterol in the blood and this causes fatty deposits which can lead to heart disease. Fat people with heart disease will reap double benefits by going on to a simple, healthy diet. Worry is the worst possible thing for anyone suffering from a heart condition and so this should be avoided wherever possible – easier said than done, I know. Any condition affecting the heart can be serious, so, if in doubt, it is wise to seek medical advice without delay. There are several excellent drugs available nowadays for the treatment of heart disease, one of the most valuable being digoxin, originally obtained from the foxglove. It strengthens the heart and slows down erratic rhythms.

H

Heart disease is the biggest single killer in Britain today. It is also a major cause of premature death. The death rate from heart disease has been dropping in many countries but to date there has been no sign of a fall in the United Kingdom. The millions of pounds spent on research have not had much success thus far.

Dr Richard Mackarness, in his book *Chemical Victims*, states: 'Professor William Rea (of USA) was elected President of the International Society for Clinical Ecology for the year 1977/78 on the strength of the work he has done on environmentally triggered disease of the heart and blood vessels.' So what are *we* doing to our food, water and air? None is pure anymore – all are polluted. Why does human health take such a low priority? Environmental factors can damage not only our hearts but all the blood vessels in our bodies. Inhaled chemicals can cause cardiac distress.

Another cause of various forms of heart condition (including angina-like pain) can be individual sensitivities to foods, food additives and chemical inhalants. A caffeine sensitivity can be provoked by taking more caffeine than the body can tolerate! We all have a caffeine threshold, varying from person to person. For some of us that means none at all! The average person may start to become aware of symptoms after perhaps five cups of coffee, depending on the strength of the coffee, the interval between each cup and other inter-related factors. The allergic, already sensitised to caffeine, may react to even a minute amount. Symptoms include palpitations (irregular heartbeat), chest pains, insomnia, anxiety, sweating, trembling, twitching, an inability to keep still and weight loss. Coffee, tea, chocolate and cola all contain caffeine as do some over-the-counter cold remedies. Watch out also for other foods to which you may have an individual sensitivity which might affect your heart. Food additives may be responsible likewise – 154 Brown FK has been implicated.

The contraceptive pill, which is a steroid, can be another precipitating factor in heart disease, especially in women over the age of thirty-five.

To sum up, therefore, preventive measures for heart conditions in general are: watch your caffeine and alcohol consumption, cut out smoking and the contraceptive pill, cut down on sugar and salt, decrease your saturated fats, exercise regularly, watch your weight, do some form of relaxation and try not to worry. Fresh fruit and fish are said to be good for the heart, and the following supplements are recommended: 1g of vitamin C daily, B complex vitamins, vitamin E (build up slowly, starting with a low dose), lecithin, dolomite (a combination of calcium and magnesium) and garlic perles.

See also **Angina** and **Chest Pains**.

HOARSENESS

In a respiratory infection the larynx may become inflamed, causing laryngitis. In a severe attack the voice will become hoarse. The condition usually lasts no longer than a week and can be relieved by inhaling steam to which *Vick* or a similar preparation has been added. If the condition does not improve, antibiotics may be required.

Allergic reactions can cause symptoms which may lead to respiratory infections – even though allergy, and not a germ, was the causative factor. The voice may become hoarse in the same manner, and the condition may require the same treatment.

Severe stress can sometimes cause a person to lose his voice or to temporarily sound husky. Take up to 3g a day of vitamin C whilst the symptoms last.

HOT FLUSHES

Hot flushes are normally associated with women going through the menopause; this usually happens when they are in their forties. The changes which take place in the hormones account for a number of unpleasant symptoms of which hot flushes are one of the most common.

As it is known that there is a definite connection between hormones and allergies, it is my belief that at any time of hormonal change a woman will find herself more susceptible to allergic reactions (or developing new allergies) than she normally would be, hence the reason for the sudden development of symptoms. If she is aware of all her allergies and is particularly careful to avoid them at this time, I see no reason why the majority of women should not get through the menopause with the minimum of symptoms.

Hot flushes are a form of sweating, and a common manifestation of a skin allergy is sweating. This can be heavy and can apply to people of any age and both sexes. There is no documentation as to the most likely causes (though plenty mentioning its existence!) with the exception of the caffeine connection, so that might be the best place to start. Caffeine is found in coffee, tea, chocolate and cola. If this does not turn up your answer then other foods will need to be considered. I have certainly observed hot flushes as a reaction to alcohol. Drugs or inhalant allergens could also be responsible. Said to be helpful for hot flushes are: vitamin E, vitamin C with bioflavonoids, B complex vitamins, selenium and ginseng.

HYPERACTIVITY (HYPERKINESIS, HYPERKINETIC SYNDROME)

Parents whose children are born with hyperactive tendencies have a very stressful and exhausting life – as do the unfortunate children themselves. That is, until the problem is recognised for what it is.

One of the more severe cases I have come across (and there are plenty of them) involved an only child called Tracy. Her parents had

H

moved to our village and bought the local sweet shop. Tracy was in her element – what six-year-old would not be! It was easy to wheedle her parents into allowing her the odd packet of Smarties or jelly babies. Soon after they arrived, Lucy, her mother, appeared one morning with pink eyes and a truly haggard expression. I asked her whatever was the matter and she told me she had walked the streets most of the night in order to 'try to use up some of my daughter's energy'. The story she told was this. Tracy was born a healthy baby. She fed well, thrived, and was no trouble until shortly after her first birthday when she became a real handful. By fourteen months she was so incessantly active that she had been put on daily sedatives to calm her down and had been taking them ever since. The trouble was that, now, on the maximum dose, she was as fidgety and restless as ever and slept only for an hour or two and then bounced around for the rest of the night allowing her parents little or no sleep. I told Lucy I thought I might be able to help – a comment she greeted with the expected scepticism. After listening to what I had to say she roared with laughter. She seemed disinclined to believe that the most usual cause of hyperactivity was artificial additives, especially the azo and coal-tar dyes so prolific in her sweet shop! I put her in touch with the Hyperactive Children's Support Group who told her the same thing. Tracy was put onto an additive-free diet and became a normal child within days. Lucy was delighted and told her doctor the sedatives were no longer needed. He was amazed at her story and has been helping hyperactive children along the same lines ever since.

Not all children are as lucky as Tracy. They may suffer from sensitivities to foods and inhalant chemicals as well as the additives in foods. They often develop eczema or asthma or other allergies at an early age in addition to the wide spectrum of symptoms possibly related to hyperactivity. As babies, they may be head-bangers or cot-rockers. (They may even be hyperactive before birth, crashing around in the womb like a team of footballers!) They are usually poor sleepers and may be poor eaters as well as they cannot sit still or concentrate long enough to get a proper meal. Some of them cry almost incessantly. As they grow older the problems worsen and they seem to be in a state of perpetual motion, are easily excitable and their behaviour is disruptive and unpredictable. Although a high IQ is as likely as in any other child, they may experience speech and learning difficulties. Balance may be a problem, causing lack of co-ordination and making them accident-prone. They are often unable to sit still for more than a few minutes, making for very poor concentration. If you are lucky they may sleep for three or four hours out of twenty-four. When they do drop off, they will be restless, talk in their sleep and suffer from nightmares. Boys are more often affected than girls, and almost all hyperactive children suffer from a constant thirst.

All this to contend with causes the most acute suffering within the family circle. Parents become desperate – especially mothers who are constantly with their child – and any social contact with relatives or friends becomes a nightmare. Mothers feel isolated and alone. They may have become social outcasts as their child causes havoc wherever he goes. He (and she) will be criticised in shops, playgroups, anywhere in fact where there is contact with other people. The mother will be blamed wherever she goes and, unless she is exceptionally lucky, by her doctor as well. Is it any wonder that this can lead to health problems, nervous breakdowns and split marriages? Because ignorance still abounds, the likelihood, even now, is that the majority of cases go undiagnosed. How much child battering, one wonders, is due to parents being driven to breaking point by this impossible situation?

Dr Ben Feingold of San Francisco was the first person in authority to realise the connection between food additives (particularly colourings and preservatives) and hyperactivity. He also believed that salicylates (found in aspirin and occurring naturally in certain fruits) were to blame. It was due to Mrs Sally Bunday sending for Dr Ben Feingold's diet, and finding that it worked so successfully for her son, that the Hyperactive Children's Support Group was born in 1977. Since then Mrs Bunday and her mother, Mrs Colquhoun, have helped thousands of families with hyperactive children return to a happy, normal life. They have given hope where the medical profession has failed.

In 1982/83 a migraine trial involving eighty-eight children was set up in Great Ormond Street Hospital for Sick Children, in London. The children, who suffered from multiple allergies, were put onto a limited diet for three to four weeks. One of the most unexpected features of the trial was the way in which other symptoms, including hyperactivity, cleared up as well (and then reappeared when the incriminating foods were reintroduced) in the great majority of children.

An international meeting of the British and American Societies for Clinical Ecology was held in Torquay in May 1984. Doctors came from all over the world and read papers on studies of food and chemical sensitivity relating to a variety of conditions including hyperactivity.

However, what does the medical profession as a whole think (with a few enlightened exceptions)? They ignore those research findings in the USA which link certain processed foods with hyperactivity and other disruptive behaviour and blame the mothers – so much easier!

What do the Government and food additive manufacturers say? They say: 'There is insufficient proof', 'the numbers are too small to be significant' or 'just leave out those foods which contain the incriminating substances.'

So, until we get the co-operation of the medical profession (head-in-sand syndrome?) and the Government (good revenue from multi-million pound processed food manufactuerers?) what can we, as individuals, do about this highly worrying situation of the steadily increasing number of hyperactive children? Prospective mothers can learn that the diet they take when pregnant plays a major role in their child's potential allergy

H

threshold. A good healthy varied diet of fresh, wholesome foods will give their unborn infant the best chance of all-round good health. When pregnant, the avoidance of drugs, wherever possible, is important but, if these should be absolutely essential, then try to ensure that they are additive-free. After your baby is born, should he/she develop colic, look to the cause (so often cow's milk) and avoid paediatric syrups which are filled with artificial colourings, flavourings and preservatives. (Boots the Chemist does a range of children's medicines which are at least free from colourings).

The 'E' numbers of colourings and preservatives which the Hyperactive Children's Support Group specifically advise against are as follows:

E102 Tartrazine	E150 Caramel
E104 Quinoline Yellow	E151 Black PN
107 Yellow 2G	154 Brown FK
E110 Sunset yellow FCF	155 Brown HT
E120 Cochineal	E210 Benzoic acid
E122 Carmosine	E211 Sodium benzoate
E123 Amaranth	E220 Sulphur dioxide
E124 Ponceau 4R	E250 Sodium nitrite
E127 Erythrosine	E249 Potassium nitrite
128 Red 2G	E251 Sodium nitrate
E132 Indigo Carmine	E320 Butylated hydroxyanisole
E133 Brilliant Blue FCF	E321 Butylated hydroxytoluene

To this list I would add E131 Patent Blue V, E142 Green S, E180 Pigment Rubine and E212 potassium benzoate (a preservative). Another preservative commonly found in fruit squashes and therefore one which causes problems over and over again is E223, sodium metabisulphite. (Why, oh why do you mothers insist upon feeding your allergic children daily with squashes containing sodium metabisulphite? What is wrong with plain water or a pure fruit juice diluted with water or soda water?)

Among other foods which may be responsible for hyperactivity and related symptoms are milk, wheat, other grains, tea, coffee, cola, citrus fruits, eggs, chocolate and sugar. Possible inhalant allergens include cleaning materials, disinfectants, floor wax, car exhaust fumes, cigarette fumes, fumes from central heating, aerosols, marker pens, perfumes, air fresheners and so on. Other likely causes are environmental pollution, nutritional and enzyme deficiencies.

What you must do is avoid giving your child processed foods (ie, food with additives), and that includes drinks as well. Buy fresh, pure foods and make your own dishes. Pulses are cheap and wholesome and are delicious cooked with gravy and a variety of vegetables. Avoid giving him caffeine – coffee, tea and cola. Cut chocolate down to a minimum. Buy sweets which do not contain colourings or preservatives, crisps which are made only from potatoes, vegetable oils and salt, and give him only water or fruit juices to drink. Check ingredients in all biscuits and cakes or (preferably) make your own. Nuts, dates, apricots (without sulphur dioxide) make good snacks, and there are some health food bars which will do nicely for his lunch box. Give him plenty of fresh fruit and vegetables. Avoid school meals if you can. It is safer to give him a packed lunch.

Many hyperactive children are found to be low in zinc. Zinc can be taken in the form of zinc sulphate or zinc gluconate. Zinc citrate is a good way to take zinc but is not suitable for anyone with a sensitivity to citric acid. Zinc gluconate seems to be more easily tolerated. It can be bought on its own or in combination with vitamin C, magnesium and the B complex vitamins. It is believed that zinc is better absorbed taken on an empty stomach last thing at night.

Some children are born sensible and mature for their years. Others cannot wait to spend their pocket money on forbidden, highly coloured sweets. My younger daughter was one of these and had to learn the hard way! They *do* learn – eventually!

It is a tremendous responsibility bringing up a hyperactive child – lonely, exhausting and, at times, heart-breaking, and a very great strain on marriages. However, as you and your child continue to work at finding out which foods, drinks and inhalants cause his symptoms, so you can expect to see his behavioural problems improve until you have them well under control.

See also **Learning Difficulties and Behaviour Problems, Hypoglycaemia.**

HYPERVENTILATION (OVER-BREATHING)

Hyperventilation means over-breathing. This causes symptoms of dizziness, light headedness, increased heart beat, lack of concentration, tiredness, tingling, or a feeling of numbness in hands, face or feet and, strangely enough, a sensation of shortness of breath.

The causes are pain (such as period pain or back pain), anxiety or sudden shock. A quick and effective means of restoring the oxygen/carbon dioxide balance is to get the patient to breathe in and out of a paper bag.

A few doctors are very hooked on hyperventilation, especially some who choose not to believe in the existence of food and chemical allergies. They believe that the over-breathing causes the symptoms. The alternative view is that the symptoms cause the over-breathing. I think one has to question why a person should over-breathe in the first place. Excluding pain and sudden shock, one is left with anxiety (see above). We can become severely anxious over events in our lives but anxiety is a common manifestation of brain allergy or sensitivity, too (experienced, for example, by someone exceeding their caffeine tolerance threshold). Patients often hyperventilate in the presence of their doctors because they are nervous and possibly do not think their doctors will believe them. Certain drugs can cause anxiety and depression and trigger over-breathing.

Hyperventilation can be caused by an adverse reaction to just about any food or chemical additive. The most obvious is caffeine-containing drinks – coffee, tea, cola and chocolate. It is worth remembering that, where a chemical inhalant is concerned, the onset of the symptoms is usually fairly rapid after exposure (whereas foods can be rapid or delayed).

Supplements recommended for anxiety would seem to be appropriate; these are: a good preparation of B complex vitamins, vitamin C, vitamin E, zinc, magnesium and calcium.

HYPOGLYCAEMIA (LOW BLOOD SUGAR)

Hypoglycaemia is, apparently, one of the most commonly undiagnosed conditions. Everybody suffers from this to some extent. It can occur for a number of reasons. Although this is still a controversial subject, all the evidence points to a correlation with food intolerance. (I do not mean that hypoglycaemia cannot have other causes but they do nearly all seem to be diet-related). The more pronounced the sensitivities, the greater the problem. In hypoglycaemia the body is unable to metabolise carbohydrates efficiently and the system over-reacts to sugar, producing too much insulin. This situation arises from two to six hours after eating.

The symptoms are faintness, irritability, lack of concentration, hunger, confusion, tiredness, and so on. If the blood sugar level falls very low, the patient may become semi-conscious or appear 'drunk' or may have epileptic-type fits. For this reason some people with food allergies have been wrongly diagnosed as epileptics. Hyperactive children can have symptoms of poor concentration and irritability due to low blood sugar. A state of hypoglycaemia is more likely to be reached after consumption of too much alcohol, tea, coffee or sweet and sugary foods. Smoking, drugs, vitamin deficiencies and stress are other aggravating factors.

Dr J C Breneman, in his book *Basics of Food Allergy*, says that it is a common clinical finding among food-intolerant people that the symptoms of hypoglycaemia appear from two to six hours after eating. Sufferers crave something sweet to return the blood sugar level to normal. Wheat allergics crave more carbohydrate. Obesity, Dr Breneman says, is often due to a recurring urge for carbohydrate.

In fact, the answer is not to go for more sugars or starches because this just sets up a vicious circle. Eat more protein and this will help to counteract the problem. Make sure you get something to eat or drink every 2–3hrs, such as an apple or carrot.

Recommended supplements are vitamins A and D, vitamin C (1g daily), vitamin E, a strong preparation of B complex vitamins, multi-minerals, kelp and acidophilus culture.

HYPOMANIA

Hypomania is described as persistent bouts of elation unrelated to circumstances. In some people it will be accompanied by alternating bouts of depression. It is a mental condition whereby the sufferer becomes euphoric and, this being so pleasant, he does not want to recognise himself as requiring treatment. His behaviour will become very odd, he may dress strangely and grossly overspend either on himself or other people. His mood may alter very rapidly, every few minutes in fact, and this extreme restlessness will cause insomnia. His behaviour is very frightening for the onlooker. He can become confused, talk a lot of nonsense, be anti-social and possibly become a danger to himself or to others. Hospital admission may become necessary.

This disorder may last for weeks or months if left untreated but the outlook is good with prompt treatment, such as lithium. The periods between attacks may last for months or even years. Although there is no generally accepted cause, the condition can be brought on by drugs. Other triggers in susceptible people may be an infection such as 'flu, the effects of alcohol, excessive worry, an intolerance to foods or a combination of any of these factors. Do not hesitate to call for immediate medical attention.

HYSTERIA

There is some controversy as to what degree of control the patient has over his own symptoms in a bout of hysteria. The general belief seems to be that the patient can sometimes increase the severity of the attack in order to gain maximum attention. A wide range of symptoms is possible. There may be an uncontrollable laughter or tears, shouts, screams, waving of arms and tearing of hair. Hysteria may resemble a fit with much writhing on the ground. On the other hand, there may be total paralysis with loss of voice, loss of sensation, loss of memory and loss of use of limbs; or any combination of these.

As shock and acute anxiety are considered to be the cause of hysteria, one would expect the patient, when recovered, to be able to give some explanation for his distress if this were not already obvious to the onlooker.

If no emotional trigger exists (or only one which would not normally warrant such acute distress) then there is the possibility of an underlying physical cause irrespective of whether or not one is actually diagnosed. One possibility is an allergic reaction to something eaten or inhaled which could cause a brain allergy so severe as to trigger a bout of hysterics. Another possibility is an imbalance of nutrients sufficient to make the individual susceptible to mood swings, making hysteria more likely. Whatever the trigger, the patient is in great distress and may need medical help.

See also **Anxiety.**

INDIGESTION

This word covers a multitude of sins! It is a generic term used to describe any upset of the normal digestive processes. It is stomach pain caused by eating too much or too fast, eating in a hurry or when you are feeling tense, or rushing up after a meal. It can also be caused by drinking too much alcohol, swallowing air whilst eating or taking foods which are too rich, too spicy or too acid. There can be serious causes, such as a peptic ulcer, and it is one of the symptoms of Crohn's disease – but these are less likely. Indigestion can also be caused by an individual food sensitivity or allergy. The best treatment is to rest and take a glass of warm water with a teaspoonful of sodium bicarbonate, whatever the cause.

Consult your doctor if symptoms increase, if there is abdominal pain, if the indigestion keeps recurring, or if you start to lose weight. If food intolerance is suspected, try to isolate the culprit by making notes of your observations. Infant indigestion is known as colic.

Magnesium, ginseng and alfalfa are all said to be natural means of helping relieve indigestion.

See also **Colic, Crohn's Disease** and **Peptic Ulcer.**

INSOMNIA (SLEEPLESSNESS)

Everyone needs sleep. It has the effect of recharging our batteries. The average adult human being is said to need eight hours, but people have different sleep requirements – some more, others less. We sleep less as we grow older. Missing sleep can make you tense, tired and irritable but, given the opportunity, you will soon catch up on this with no ill effects.

So what about the inability to sleep? Many people tend to worry unnecessarily about this, thus keeping themselves awake all the more! You are still resting your body even if you are awake. We need to feel comfortable in our bodies and minds in order to relax and make sleep possible. A strange environment, too much heat, cold, light or noise will disturb our sleep pattern – as will illness or irregular hours, such as shift workers have to get used to.

One of the hardest things about being the mother of a new baby is the loss of sleep owing to the need to provide nightly feeds. It requires the most tremendous effort – at a time when you most need your sleep – but luckily Nature has endowed mothers with a strong instinct to attend to their baby's needs, and babies with the most adequate means of making their needs known!

The most common causes of sleeplessness (or alternatively, early waking) are an overstimulated mind, worry, or depression. It is not always easy to do something about this situation even when we know the cause. However, it so often happens that when events unfold we find we have been worrying unnecessarily!

However, if you have not got anything on your mind and there is nothing in your surroundings to disturb you then you must look else-where for the cause of your insomnia. You could be reacting to a food or inhalant. Insomnia is one of the most common mental symptoms of food intolerance.

The most likely culprit is caffeine – a known stimulant. It is not sufficient to say 'I do not drink coffee (tea/chocolate) before I go to bed', because the effects can last much longer than that. Neither does it help to say 'I drink only X number of cups of coffee a day' because your own individual caffeine tolerance level could be lower than this, perhaps even nil!

Sleeping pills are not advisable on a regular basis because you can become addicted to them. Their effects can last into your working hours which, if you drive to work, could be dangerous. They can react badly with other drugs and should not be taken with alcohol.

I would recommend all pill-popping insomniacs to give up their sleeping pills and their caffeine at the same time. They could be very surprised at how well they are sleeping in less than a week! If caffeine is not responsible, then other foods may be to blame.

So what else will help? A good bed is the first essential – then there is daily exercise and, before bed, a hot bath and a warm drink (milk is ideal if you can tolerate it). Reading in bed is very relaxing too.

Taking B vitamins and dolomite (calcium and magnesium) will help to induce sleep.

IRRITABILITY

Irritability is natural in all of us at times – worry, depression, fear, anxiety, tension (not to mention other people's behaviour!) can all cause us to feel irritable, and it is not always easy to control.

Irritability is also a symptom of diabetes, hypoglycaemia, insomnia and pre-menstrual syndrome (PMS). It is one of the milder symptoms of schizophrenia and other medical conditions. It can be caused by the effects of caffeine or a side-effect of drugs. It can also be due to a lack of B vitamins, especially B1, and B12 or vitamin C or iron (anaemia). It is a well established symptom of asthma, hay fever and hyperactivity and accompanies colic in babies.

Other causes of irritability are allergies to foods, chemicals in foods, and inhalants (such as gas). Any food can be responsible – cow's milk is a likely one. It is a common reaction to food additives (one of the main triggers in hyperactivity).

The B vitamins, vitamin C, manganese and the amino acids trypto-phan and tyrosine will all help to stabilise the temperament. Extra iron is essential if the patient is found to be anaemic.

See also **Hypoglycaemia, Premenstrual Syndrome.**

IRRITABLE BOWEL SYNDROME (SPASTIC COLON/IRRITABLE COLON)

Irritable bowel syndrome is a very common condition. It usually starts affecting people under the age of thirty, and it affects twice as many women as men. The name is a generic term for a variety of different bowel problems which commonly involve diarrhoea but may involve constipation or alternating bouts of both. There can be a severe ache over the lower colon (lower left abdomen) and in many cases there is distension or bloating of the stomach. Other symptoms which may be present are mucus in the stool, lack of concentration, fatigue, depression and anxiety. There may be a tendency to urinate more often. Irritable bowel syndrome can last from days to months and, if the cause is not isolated, can continue for many years.

The advice given by the orthodox medical profession regarding diet is usually limited to taking extra fibre in the form of bran. This may be useful where constipation is concerned but is quite unhelpful when the patient is suffering from diarrhoea (especially if he turns out to be wheat sensitive!). Other orthodox advice is to recommend 'plenty of exercise', 'try to relax' and 'avoid stressful situations'. (What more stressful situation than suffering from irritable bowel syndrome?) They may also treat the patient with drugs for anxiety and depression which, as a long-term solution, is best avoided.

It is true that the less dietary fibre eaten the greater the risk of bowel disease. However, wheat bran is not the only bran – there is soya bran and rice bran. Neither is bran the only fibre. Other whole grains, raw fruit and raw or lightly cooked vegetables are all good sources to anyone eating a natural, healthy, balanced diet should not even have to worry.

Irritable bowel syndrome frequently starts after a bout of gastroenteritis or after repeated courses of antibiotics. Both of these cause changes in the bacteria lining the intestines. Research by Dr John Hunter of Addenbrooke's Hospital, Cambridge, shows that IBS patients may have a disturbed gut flora. The diarrhoea or antibiotics may have removed the beneficial flora allowing the unwanted bacteria to produce toxins which could trigger reactions to specific foods. Two major trials of IBS patients by Dr John Hunter and Dr Virginia Alun Jones were carried out at Addenbrooke's Hospital, showing that the majority of patients were food intolerant and improved considerably when the identified foods were removed from their diets.

In other trials, which have not been so successful, the reason may have been that wheat (one of the most common causes of IBS) was not always excluded. Another reason may have been that small amounts of food were given at the time of challenge; in some patients much larger amounts are required, or the same food must be eaten over a period of days before the symptoms return.

The only alternative that the non-food-intolerance brigade can come up with is that this illness is psychosomatic – basing their view on the symptoms of anxiety and depression and the fact that X-rays and blood tests are always normal. (The same reasoning applies equally to food intolerance, however. Depression and anxiety are common manifestations of allergic reaction. Of course the blood tests are negative because they are not testing for food allergies!)

Can you imagine how depressing it must be to have your life dominated by continuous diarrhoea? Can you also imagine how anxious it would make you to be told that the action of your own mind is causing your physical symptoms. To be anxious and depressed in these circumstances, I suggest, is *normal*. To be totally unconcerned – now that *would* suggest the need to question someone's mental state! Also, the allergens implicated in IBS are as likely to affect the brain as the gut.

Once the patient has developed the problem there are various factors which will aggravate the symptoms – including menstrual changes, lack of fibre, stress and so on, but these are *not* the cause. The cause is most likely to be food intolerances, although enzyme deficiencies may be involved. Either way it is most important for the patient to discover which foods are causing these distressing symptoms. Any foods or drinks may be involved. Among the most common are wheat, corn, cow's milk and its products, eggs, cheese, coffee, tea and citrus fruits. Food additives are frequently incriminated in IBS. Watch out particularly for E110, E131, E132, E210, E221–E227, E239, E250, E252, E282, E310–E312, E406, E407, E421, 430, E450(b), E450(c), 503, 508, 545, 621, 924.

For recommended supplements see entries dealing with individual symptoms: **Abdominal Pain, Anxiety, Bloating, Constipation, Depression, Diarrhoea, Fatigue** and **Indigestion**.

There is so much you can do to help yourself. Start by putting yourself onto an elimination diet. You really *can* get well again!

KIDNEY DISORDERS

We are born with two kidneys. They serve the purpose of filtering the blood and depositing the waste products into the urine.

Kidney diseases are important because they can lead to kidney failure. If the kidneys fail to remove the toxic waste products from our blood, then artificial kidney machines must be used instead. The machines can sometimes be installed in people's own homes. It is a time-consuming and costly business and not very pleasant for the patient who may benefit more from a transplant. We can help by becoming kidney donors.

Kidney stones (which are hard masses of mineral salts) can form in any part of the urinary tract, including the kidneys or bladder. They can be caused by either a blood abnormality or an infection. They may be due to an over-consumption of, or individual reaction to, sugars. Professor Norman Blacklock of Manchester University Medical School has done a study linking processed sugars in foods with kidney stones.

The people most at risk of developing kidney disorders are the young and the elderly. Newly married and pregnant women can develop infections causing back pain and fever. People with high blood pressure, diabetes and allergies are also susceptible to kidney disorders.

The following symptoms are all possible indications of kidney disorders: back pain, fluid retention, swelling – especially in face, arms, legs and ankles, a burning sensation when passing urine, frequent urination, possible bed-wetting in children, and a raised temperature. Medical advice should be sought anyway, but the matter is urgent if there is severe pain in the kidney area, blood in the urine or an inability to pass urine.

Certain precautions can be taken in order to help prevent urinary tract infections and kidney disorders. Observe normal measures of genital hygiene (women are advised to wipe themselves from front to back in order to avoid infecting the bladder). Do not exceed recommended doses of aspirin and other pain-killers as excessive doses can damage the kidneys. Conversely, people with kidney disease have to be very careful about taking drugs because of impaired excretion leading to toxic build-up.

Kidney disorders are normally caused by factors unrelated to allergy, but certain foods can cause kidney damage in some people. Nephritis, or inflammation of the kidneys, is a very serious condition, and cow's milk and pork have been reported as proven causes of this. Pollens and other airborne allergens have also been linked with kidney disorders.

One of the treatments for allergies known as auto-immune urine therapy (which means injecting the patient with his own sterilised urine) can be extremely damaging to the kidneys as it can cause the immune system to start fighting off its own tissue.

A magnesium supplement is an effective deterrent against developing kidney stones (especially useful if taking a daily vitamin C supplement) as it helps to prevent the build-up of mineral deposits. See also **Cystitis**.

LACK OF LIBIDO (SEXUAL DEFICIENCY)

Living with anyone requires compromises in all directions, and the physical relationship is no exception. Despite a wide difference of sexual appetites, most couples manage to reach a satisfactory compromise.

However, if one partner is feeling weak, ill, fatigued and struggling to get through the day (all classic symptoms of allergic reaction) this does not make for a very satisfactory sex life. In addition, allergies can actually *cause* lack of libido, frigidity and impotence.

A number of women develop their first allergic symptoms after starting the Pill, which is a steroid, a fact which is seldom mentioned. Dr Ellen Grant has linked migraine and other allergies with the contraceptive pill whilst working in the migraine department of London's Charing Cross Hospital in the 1970s. Very little is known of its long-term effects.

To put it quite simply: you have to be feeling well to have any desire for a physical relationship, irrespective of how much you love your partner.

Some people believe that vitamin E improves libido, although no official studies have been done. It has, however, been shown to improve the reproductive abilities of female rats, so make of that what you will. Personally I recommend it. It is officially recommended for pregnant or lactating women, women on the Pill, women over forty, and anyone else who feels they could do with rejuvenating. A strong preparation of B complex vitamins, zinc and ginseng may all help in this direction too.

See also **the Pill**.

LACTASE DEFICIENCY (LACTOSE INTOLERANCE)

Lactose is milk sugar. It is found in the milk of mammals. We need an enzyme, lactase, in order to digest the lactose. Some people do not produce this enzyme – or they produce too little. In general terms, Mediterranean, Asian and black people have lower amounts of lactase than people of European origin. The symptoms of lactase deficiency are pain, diarrhoea and wind.

Very occasionally, babies are lacking in this enzyme; this means that they are unable to tolerate either their mother's milk or cow's milk. As they will be made very ill by either, they will need to be fed on one of the brands of soya milk designed especially for babies. These contain no lactose as they come from a bean and not a mammary gland. Some babies, although able to produce lactase, have insufficient to cope with large feeds – which may account for *some* cases of infant colic.

Being milk sensitive is another matter altogether. It is not unusual for babies intolerant to milk to be classified as lactase deficient when, in fact, the majority are allergic to cow's milk and are reacting to the proteins in it. It is not always easy to differentiate between the two conditions, but lactose-intolerant babies will be made very ill by either cow's milk or breast milk, and milk-intolerant babies will probably show some other symptoms instead of, or in addition to, the pain, diarrhoea and wind of the enzyme-deficient babies. These symptoms are likely to be either eczema, asthma, croup, constipation or ear allergy (serous otitis). A milk-allergic baby will thrive well on breast milk if the mother is on a dairy-free diet herself or, alternatively, on a soya-based formula.

For the rest, some of us will lose this enzyme as we grow into childhood or adulthood and therefore taking any milk will cause us these same symptoms. Certain milk products such as yoghurt and cheese are better tolerated because they contain far less lactose. (But then, a milk-*allergic* person can regain a tolerance to certain milk products too!) Whether it is a lactase deficiency or milk allergy, it is much the same as far as the patient is concerned. If you want to stay well give up milk! It is not as if the medical profession has some magical answer to either.

A lactase deficiency occurs in everyone on a *temporary* basis following a bout of diarrhoea (for whatever reason) as our internal digestive systems need a recovery period before being able to produce sufficient lactase again. If milk is consumed at this time, then the diarrhoea could start up again. Therefore, the golden rule, which applies to adults and children alike, is: leave milk out of your diet for a few days (or as long as it takes) following an attack of gastroenteritis or other tummy upset.

Watch out for lactose in many medicines and some supplements where it is used as a sweetener. For recommended supplements look under individual symptoms. See **Abdominal Pain, Colic, Diarrhoea, Indigestion.**

LEARNING DIFFICULTIES AND BEHAVIOUR PROBLEMS

I well remember as a child an occasion when, being helped with my maths homework, my father asked me (getting fairly desperate by this time) what one per cent of a hundred was. I was unable to answer him and he was none too pleased. I tell this anecdote to illustrate how some children have, at times, great difficulty in getting their brains to function *at all*. This applies to adults as well, of course, and obviously there are many varied reasons why this should happen: physical illness, shock, distress, overwork and so on.

However, those people who are subject to brain allergies are at a great disadvantage. It is generally recognised now by doctors working in this field that certain foods and food additives act like drugs on such people. This I can most certainly confirm from personal experience!

With regard to the effect of chemical inhalants, these people may have a low toxic threshold. In other words, the concentration of a chemical deemed safe for general use may affect them one hundred times more than it might affect someone else.

Children suffer the most because they are least able to make themselves understood and they often have to pay a severe penalty for their 'stupidity'.

An allergic child may have learning problems due to hearing difficulties which come and go with food exposures. He may suffer adverse reactions to the cheap, strong-smelling chemical disinfectants used to clean his school or the scented toiletries used in his home. He may be exposed to many different allergens in the course of a day.

Any, or several, of the following symptoms may be exhibited by the typically allergic child: short concentration span, restlessness, aggressiveness, over-activity, excitability, difficulting in relating to peers, constantly fidgeting, constantly demanding attention, easily frustrated, tearful, rapid mood changes, outbursts of temper, nervousness, anxiety, listlessness, perpetual tiredness. These children are usually pale, with dark circles under their eyes and a general appearance of ill-health. They may have an intense thirst and/or suffer from headaches. My own view is that maybe one in five children is predisposed this way. Certainly one in ten would be a conservative estimate.

A child who suffers from brain allergies, however, is likely to have (or have had) other symptoms which are more easily recognised as allergic – such as asthma, eczema or gut problems. Many of these children will improve beyond recognition when put onto an additive-free diet which excludes coloured sweets, squashes, fizzy drinks, flavoured snacks and other foods or drinks which contain chemical additives. Others may need to go onto an elimination diet – likely culprit include cow's milk, wheat, oranges, cheese, chocolates, eggs, peanuts, sugar, tea, coffee and pork.

See also **Hyperactivity**.

LOSS OF SENSE OF SMELL AND TASTE

Some people are born with a poor sense of smell. Presumably our taste buds also vary in their ability to function. We lose our sense of smell when we have colds, catarrh, sinusitis and similar afflictions. To a certain extent our sense of taste is diminished then also. None of this worries us too much as we know it is only temporary. It is an added burden, however, to the all-year-round hayfever sufferer. He also runs the fairly minor risk of developing nasal polyps as a result of prolonged irritation to the nasal membranes. These can cause a loss of sense of smell but, if they are troublesome, they can be surgically removed quite easily.

Some people find they have lost their sense of taste and smell *completely* and this, by all accounts, seems to cause much distress. I should not rule out the possibility of an allergy but the most likely reason for this may be a dietary deficiency. A balanced diet – including foods rich in potassium, B vitamins, biotin and calcium – should help. Many people find that they are low on zinc, and so a zinc supplement along with additional Vitamin A can often restore the lost senses. For loss of smell, Earl Mindell (in *The Vitamin Bible*) recommends 50mg chelated zinc three times daily – one to two times daily when the condition improves.

See also **Hay Fever** and **Nasal Polyps**.

MALNUTRITION

People who are undernourished are described as suffering from malnutrition. This term applies equally to people who may be getting enough to eat but who are on a diet with insufficient nutrients to sustain good health and growth. There is yet another group of people who suffer from malnutrition; they are the ones who have difficulty in *absorbing* the nutrients in their food – for example, children suffering from coeliac disease cannot absorb their food properly as a result of intestinal damage caused by intolerance to the gluten in wheat, oats, barley and rye. When food cannot properly be absorbed, malnutrition results. After gluten has been removed from their diets, they thrive normally.

Coeliac disease is, however, only one example. Some people suffer from malnutrition through unrecognised food intolerances causing malabsorption. In fact such people produce stools in which the foods eaten have passed through the system to be evacuated in apparently the same form as when they were consumed.

Diarrhoea is a common symptom of food intolerance. When young children suffer from it these days doctors tend to say 'It is only "toddler diarrhoea" – he will grow out of it.' There never used to be such a thing as 'toddler diarrhoea', and a child whose weight gain is poor through suffering constant diarrhoea is at risk of developing malnutrition; a malnourished child is susceptible to disease and to the development of more allergies. Someone found to be suffering from malnutrition needs to be put onto a fresh, wholesome diet of foods which they can tolerate.

Doctors are taught very little about nutrition, and some choose 'not to believe in' food allergies in spite of the fact that there have been articles on the subject published in the *Lancet* and other medical journals for many years now. Nutrition is a matter for dieticians – they are the specialists – but they may have little knowledge or understanding of food allergies. Patients are forced to look elsewhere for help. Many of the therapists to whom they turn know little more. A number have put their patients at risk by putting them on such restricted diets that they are short of essential nutrients for *long periods of time*. Children are particularly vulnerable because they need extra nutrients for growth.

It suits some doctors to say that diets are dangerous. This needs to be clarified. Some are. However, an elimination diet of the type advocated in this book (see Chapter 5) is of foods which are natural and nutritious (you can eat as much as you want as often as you want) and it specifies that the diet should not be used for longer than a maximum of two weeks before re-introducing other foods. A diet such as this is quite safe.

It is *after* you have sorted out your food allergies that you need the expertise of a dietician to ensure that you are getting a balanced diet. What is so essential for all of us is that we get a varied diet of pure, natural foods to provide us with the necessary nutrients. If you find that you cannot tolerate something, there is always something else with which it can be substituted. Don't be fooled by processed foods which are advertised as having extra vitamins and minerals added. They probably lost most of their natural ones whilst being processed! Some will contain chemical additives of which the long-term effects are not yet known. Poor nutrition decreases our resistance to stress. A well-nourished person is far better equipped to face the ups and downs of this hazardous and unpredictable world in which we live.

A strong vitamin and mineral supplement will help everyone to reach their own health potential.

See also **Coeliac Disease** and **Toddler Diarrhoea**.

MÉNIÈRE'S DISEASE

Ménière's disease is a condition of the inner ear which affects the balance. It is caused by congestion which may be inflammatory or allergic in origin. It does not occur in children. It was first described by a French physician, Prosper Ménière, in the last century, and in 1921 Dr William Duke of Kansas City published a report in which he produced evidence that it could be caused by food allergies.

The symptoms include sudden vertigo (dizziness), nausea or vomiting, headaches, pallor and possible disturbances of hearing and vision. It usually involves only one ear but in a small number of cases both ears will be affected. Attacks can start suddenly and the patient will need to go to bed. For a few hours the symptoms may be very severe. If a doctor needs to be called he will probably give an injection or prescribe medication. The frequency and severity of attacks are likely to increase unless the cause is found. The cause nearly always turns out to be an adverse reaction to a food or drink (or even medicine). By writing down everything you have eaten and drunk over the twenty-four hours *prior* to an attack, and comparing notes after two or three times, a common factor should emerge; otherwise, an elimination diet will help.

Niacin, one of the B vitamins, known variously as nicotinic acid, niacinamide or nicotinamide, is said to help reduce the distressing symptom of vertigo.

See also **Tinnitus**.

M

MENOPAUSE (THE CHANGE OF LIFE)

The menopause, which means a gradual slowing down and stopping of the menstrual cycle, usually occurs in women somewhere between the ages of forty and fifty-five. The changes are not necessarily abrupt and may continue over a period of time, although all women will vary. When a woman reaches the change of life she loses her ability to conceive children, but contraceptives should be used until the change is complete and then a sexual relationship can continue unfettered by worries of pregnancy.

Any vaginal dryness can be helped with the use of KY jelly. Some women may need an oestrogen cream prescribed by their doctor. Others will benefit from hormone replacement therapy (HRT) but this involves having to return to the monthly period. It helps with the symptoms but is not suited to everyone as it does carry some risks and can trigger off migraines in certain people (as can the Pill).

During the change there may be some weight gain due to hormonal changes. For the same reason some women suffer certain unpleasant symptoms. The more common ones are hot flushes, sweating, depression, insomnia, fatigue and headache.

There is no doubt that the menopause, just like any other hormonal change, is linked to allergy. It lowers a woman's allergy threshold making her more susceptible than usual to allergic reactions. By discovering and eliminating the food and inhalant allergens which trigger off the symptoms, women can go through the change virtually symptom-free.

Let me give you an example. I have a friend who broke out in a sweat every time she drank gin. She put it down to the change and she was right inasmuch as this had not happened before she started the menopause but it was certainly *triggered* by the gin as I observed with fascination every lunch time during her stay with us. Had she been prepared to relinquish her gin, even on a temporary basis, she might have been able to return to it later on with no ill effects.

Conversely, many symptoms of allergy (migraine is a good example) which have previously been triggered or aggravated by the monthly period will disappear after the menopause is over.

There is a loss of calcium from the bones during this time so this should be supplemented. Calcium combined with magnesium in the form of dolomite is a good way. Other recommended supplements are vitamin E, vitamin C (1g daily), selenium, a strong preparation of B complex vitamins and ginseng.

For further information on HRT contact the Amarant Trust; address at back of book.

See also **Menstruation**.

MENSTRUATION (PERIODS)

The womb lining undergoes a monthly cycle of hormonal changes in preparation for receiving a fertilised egg. If none is forthcoming the blood-stained lining is discharged and this is known as menstruation or a period. If conception occurs then periods stop. Girls can start menstruating any time from ten until well into their teens (the average age being around twelve or thirteen) and they will continue with monthly periods until they reach the change of life, probably in their forties or fifties.

Occasionally periods can stop for reasons other than conception, and missing the odd one is of no consequence, but if they are continually missed then it would be sensible to go and have a chat with your doctor. The failure to menstruate is known as amenorrhoea and is seldom serious. Assuming that you are sure there is no chance of your being pregnant, and you are not going through even an early menopause, your doctor will check on the possibility of any form of illness. If he is unable to give any explanation, do remember this: if you are on the Pill, which is a steroid, the Pill will interfere with the body's natural functions and can cause hormonal side-effects which may be the root of your loss of periods. Discuss this with your doctor.

Sometimes just before or at the start of a period there is pain in the lower abdomen or backache or both. Menstrual cramps are not uncommon. A small number of women suffer more than most; they turn very pale and need to go to bed with a hot water bottle and some pain-killers for twenty-four hours. This painful menstruation is called dysmenorrhoea.

Extra heavy periods can occur from time to time and, whilst being a nuisance, are no real problem. If they should become frequent, then this is known as menorrhagia and medical advice should be sought as you may need extra iron to prevent you from becoming anaemic. Similarly, if you start to pass large clots of blood on a regular basis you run the risk of becoming anaemic and may need extra iron.

All these abnormal forms of menstruation and the more commonplace (but sometimes very distressing) pre-menstrual syndrome have a number of different causes and these should be investigated. Sometimes allergy to foods, chemicals in foods or inhalants is the root cause. Some women find that they are sensitive only to certain foods just before or at the start of a period. If they avoid them at this time they find that they can sail through their period with a minimum of symptoms. These foods may be able to be consumed at other times without ill-effect. Such people suffer from borderline allergies which need a final trigger to set them in motion.

Other gynaecological problems may be caused by food allergies. It is always necessary to have these checked out first by your doctor, or a gynaecologist if necessary, but it is worth remembering that if no other cause can be found foods may be responsible. Milk and eggs are the most likely because you are introducing a *foreign* female protein into your body.

Recommended supplements are vitamin K (menadione) – natural sources yoghurt and alfalfa tablets – for menorrhagia; vitamin A and zinc for amenorrhoea. For dysmenorrhoea, pre-menstrual syndrome and general menstrual symptoms, take Oil of Evening Primrose, a strong preparation of B complex vitamins and extra B6. Dolomite (calcium and magnesium) is said to be helpful too. All menstruating women are at risk of becoming anaemic so they may need to take extra iron. Menstruating women who are vegetarians are especially at risk, but a simple blood test in the surgery can put your mind at rest on this score.

See also **Menopause, the Pill** and **Pre-menstrual Syndrome** (PMS).

M

MENTAL CONFUSION

Dr Albert Rowe of California, who started working in the field of allergy after the First World War, pioneered the elimination diet in the treatment of food allergy symptoms. He proved that it could alleviate a variety of chronic symptoms – including mental ones – and that these same symptoms would return when incriminating foods were re-introduced. In other words, he proved that foods could be responsible for mental illness. Add to that the introduction of food additives and chemical pollutants and you get a vast increase in potential allergens! The introduction of North Sea gas in people's homes has proved to be another possible hazard. All these are proven causes of allergic reaction in susceptible people – of whom the numbers are ever on the increase – and where the allergy affects the brain, mental symptoms will result. These are wide-ranging, but the ones associated with mental confusion are memory loss, inability to assimilate facts, difficulty in following a routine, inability to comprehend or communicate. To an observer this may be just an interesting phenomenon. To the sufferer it is a terrifying and bewildering nightmare. He desperately needs your help and understanding.

I cannot over-emphasise the need to discover the offending items, but in order to help counteract the mental confusion you should also take a strong preparation of vitamin B complex, vitamin C (1g daily), vitamin E, zinc and dolomite.

See also **Brain Allergies**.

MENTAL ILLNESS

Mental illness is a vast subject covering many different conditions with innumerable reasons for them. One person in seven is expected to suffer some form of mental illness in their lives and I suspect many more do but it goes unrecognised. Most people veer between normal and abnormal throughout their lifetime – it is a question of degree. In any case, are the ones who make the classification qualified to do so? Certainly, if there is a consensus of opinion that the behaviour of the person in question is causing concern or has become decidedly anti-social. However, *everyone* has a breaking point if sufficient pressure is applied – it is really a matter of how many pressures converge on us at any given time.

Mental illness can be caused by brain dysfunction, physical illness, circumstances, emotional disturbances, an unbalanced mind, too many pressures, hormone imbalance, mental suffering, the effects of alcohol, the Pill or other drugs, stressful relationships and many other things. Over some of these situations we have control and it is essential that we use this control where we can for the sake of others and for self-preservation.

Chemical imbalance is something over which we have control *only* when we understand the problem. Conditions such as diabetes and thyroid malfunction can cause mental symptoms at times which can, in the main, be stabilised. The same applies to sensitivity to medical drugs, caffeine, foods, food additives and chemical inhalants. If we know what we are up against we stand a good chance of avoiding them. The tragedy is that there are many people confined to mental hospitals under doctors who have no knowledge of the effects of sensitivities on the individual and have no desire to take into account the observations of their patients' relatives. The effects of alcohol are the only exception to this.

The foods most likely to be associated with allergies causing mental symptoms are wheat, milk, coffee, tea, sugar, eggs and pork.

A woman I know suffered from such severe depression that she slashed her wrists and was taken into her local mental hospital. Luckily she survived the ordeal. She came to the conclusion that wheat was the cause of her depression but, as no one was interested in her observations, she was served wheat with every meal. She discharged herself, came to see me, went onto a wheat-free diet, suffered a period of withdrawal and finally emerged a happy lady. On a wheat-free diet she has remained well ever since. How many others, I wonder?

Chemical sensitivities can cause depression and other mental symptoms too. Just about any chemical can be involved. Suspect first those with which you come into regular contact, either at your place of work or in or around your own home.

See also **Brain Allergies, Mental Confusion** and **Schizophrenia**.

M

MENTAL RETARDATION (MENTAL SUBNORMALITY)

Mental retardation is the name for all conditions where the brain has not developed normally. There are varying degrees of retardation and some people may be more intelligent in one respect than another. An average IQ is a hundred, and anything below eighty is usually considered subnormal.

There are some excellent schools and centres around for mentally handicapped children, and it is important that if you have a child with this problem he should be given the advantage of their experience and expertise to help him reach his full potential.

At the same time, it is essential to try to discover why your child appears to be mentally handicapped in case anything can be done. There has to be a reason. Was it a very difficult birth? Could he have sustained an injury at this time? Might he have inherited a genetic abnormality? Is there any history of this on either side of the family? If the answer is 'yes' to any of these questions, there is still much which can be done. Find out about schools for the mentally handicapped in your area. Do they have a pre-school or nursery unit? Get him entered as soon as possible. Many of the teachers in such schools have experience and dedication which is quite remarkable. The sooner he takes advantage of this, the more they will be able to do for him.

If your answer was 'no' to the above questions, then consider the following: could your child be suffering from lack of nutrients? I do not mean to suggest that you have not fed him correctly, but a diet deficient in essential fatty acids can harm the brain and central nervous system. Any child living on a diet of processed foods who, in addition, consumes a fair amount of coloured sweets, coloured squashes and flavoured snacks is at risk here. Could he be suffering from vitamin and mineral deficiencies caused by a malabsorption problem? (See Malnutrition.) Has he ever been exposed to toxic heavy metals, (lead, mercury, cadmium, etc) or were you whilst pregnant?

If your answer is 'no' to all these questions, and no one in the medical profession has been able to give you a satisfactory explanation for his poor mental development, I suggest you consider the possibility of food or chemical allergies. Is there a family history of allergy? (Even if the answer is 'no' here, I would point out that food and chemical sensitivity is on the increase, and more babies are being born with this problem than in the past.) Did he develop satisfactorily in the early stages? If so, then try to think back to the time when his progress started to slow down or stop. Might it relate to the time of his weaning? Did you notice a change in him when first introducing him to cow's milk or to any new solids? Did he have an illness or trauma from which you can relate his lack of development? If his responses were within normal limits to start with but his progress stopped at some *later* stage, then there *has* to be a reason for it. Because this is not always taken into account, some children are wrongly diagnosed as being mentally retarded *when they are actually sensitive to foods or chemicals*. Do foods, in these instances, cause the allergic reactions, or are the reactions due to a pharmacological response causing the foods to act like drugs? We know either can be the case but this, whilst being of interest, is not relevant as far as getting the child back to normal is concerned.

What needs to be done is for him to be put onto an elimination diet (see Chapter 5) – at the same time removing from his environment all possible inhalant allergens (see Introduction). I hope very much that you will see an improvement in him within a week. Sometimes it takes a little longer but you should see some results within two weeks and I should not continue the diet for more than a maximum of three weeks. As soon as you notice a marked improvement start re-introducing his usual foods, one at a time, monitoring as you go, to see which ones are the culprits. Common causes are milk, wheat, eggs, artificial additives (particularly colourings, preservatives and citric acid) and chemical inhalants.

Whatever the cause, all retarded children benefit from taking high potency vitamin and mineral supplements (never exceeding the stated dose) because these will help them to reach their full potential.

See also **Brain Allergies**, and **Learning Difficulties and Behaviour Problems**.

MIGRAINE

Migraine is one of the most common diseases of the nervous system. Five per cent of the population is said to suffer from migraines, and women are more prone to them than men. The tendency often runs in families. Most migraine sufferers are susceptible to ordinary headaches and other allergy-induced symptoms too.

The initial symptoms of migraine are a premonition that one is about to start and a headache, and possibly nausea, accompanied by any of the following: disturbed vision, numbness, tingling of hands and feet, dizziness, confusion, weakness, and possible difficulty with speech. These symptoms can be summed up as general disorientation, feeling very groggy, and a feeling of being cut off from the rest of humanity. As if this were not enough, it will be followed by a severe, throbbing headache, nausea or vomiting and the need to remove oneself from the light.

Anyone who has experienced this will know that the only thing to do is to lie down in a darkened room, take pain-killers, wait for the worst to pass and pray that everyone will leave you in peace. These distressing symptoms can last from a few hours up to several days. The migraine has to work itself through before the sufferer can begin to return to anything like normal. Aspirin, codeine and paracetamol are the usual choice of pain-killer to relieve the headache.

The first symptoms are caused by the narrowing of the blood vessels leading to one side of the head. The very severe headache follows when the arteries widen again. This is known as 'classical migraine'. In so-called 'cluster migraines' one suffers from one migraine after another in a short space of time, interspersed with long migraine-free periods.

Children can suffer from migraine in a slightly different form. They are more likely to experience pain in the abdomen which may or may not be accompanied by a headache. This is known as 'abdominal migraine'. Any of the following symptoms may also be present with abdominal migraine, confirming the fact that allergy is likely to be the root cause: diarrhoea, wind, hyperactivity, aching limbs, runny nose, mouth ulcers, asthma, eczema and vaginal discharge.

There are many different triggers of migraine, and people learn to avoid those which are avoidable. However, several studies have been done which show that an underlying allergy to a common food or inhalant is often *the major cause*, lowering the patient's allergy threshold so that it takes only a relatively minor trigger to set a migraine in motion. These basic causes can be discovered by going onto an elimination diet where they will reveal themselves in no uncertain terms during the reintroduction procedure.

The most common basic allergens in migraine responsible for lowering the patient's allergy threshold are alcohol, (especially red wine and champagne), milk, eggs, wheat, corn, oranges, cheese (especially

M

Cheddar), chocolate, coffee, tea, beef, cane sugar, yeast, nuts, tomatoes, mushrooms, peas, peanuts, pork, fish and food additives. The food additives most frequently incriminated are E102 tartrazine, E210 benzoic acid, E281 sodium propionate, E282 calcium propionate, 621 monosodium glutamate, 622 monopotassium glutamate and 623 calcium glutamate. Watch out for individual reactions to any other additives.

Likely chemical inhalants are perfumes, exhaust fumes, pesticides, gas, oil, formaldehyde and cigarette smoke. Occasionally, non-chemical inhalants such as house dust and pollens can be responsible.

Migraine specialists often ask people to exclude a single well-documented food allergen then, when the migraines do not clear up, conclude that food allergy is not to blame. They are not taking into account the fact that patients are likely to be sensitive to more than one food, and possibly to inhalants as well, in which case this method of testing can never be conclusive. It is no substitution for a properly monitored elimination diet conducted in conjunction with the consideration of possible inhalant allergens as well.

Adverse reactions to alcohol are hardly ever to the alcohol itself (unless people have over-indulged) but are much more likely to be to the constituents such as wheat, barley, sugar, yeast etc. These foods, in soluble form, are more potent and are rapidly absorbed into the blood stream, thereby causing reactions which can appear quite rapidly. An addicted beer or whisky drinker may, in fact, be a wheat addict! The migraine arrives only when he stops!

Some people are sensitive to vegetable gums which are present in medicines, cosmetics, sweets and newspaper print, as well as foods. Others may suffer a sugar allergy/addiction, and some people believe that too much salt can cause migraines.

In addition to allergic reactions there are further problems. Cheese and chocolate contain phenylethlamine, a substance to which the blood vessels are sensitive. There are some people who lack certain enzymes. Monoamine oxidase, for example, is the enzyme required to break down the amino acid tyramine, which is present in red wine, cheeses, chicken livers, pickled herrings, cured meats, caviar, chocolate, yoghurt, broad beans and some beers. Tyramine causes the blood vessels in the head to swell.

The onset of migraine (and/or headaches) may start in some women after they have been prescribed the Pill. The contraceptive pill is a steroid and it alters a woman's hormone balance. Cigarettes contain chemicals which alter the body's chemistry, so smoking (or inhaling other people's smoke) can be a cause of migraine also. Commonly prescribed medication for migraine sufferers are tablets containing ergotamine tartrate, and patients can become sensitised to them as a result of regular exposure; thus, these tablets can become a cause of migraine too. Ergotamine should *never* be taken by a pregnant woman.

So, these are the possible causes. There may be a lurking migraine as a result of any one of them. It needs only a trigger to act as 'the last straw' to set the migraine in motion. Such triggers are fatigue, worry, bright or flashing lights, noise, extremes of temperature, pre-menstrual syndrome, overwork, emotional stress and so on. Migraines can be activated by flickering lights, and even television can be enough to affect some people. Overwork, exercise, emotional stress or the time *following stress* can all act as triggers too. Surprisingly, over sleeping has been named too.

Women often complain of attacks of migraine just before or just after menstruation has started but, time and time again, after being put on the right track, they have found a food, drink or inhalant to be the *cause* of the migraine and their period only a *trigger*. Migraine often ceases completely after the menopause for this reason.

People who experience weekend migraines are usually suffering delayed reactions to (or withdrawal symptoms from) something experienced during the week but not at weekends. (Withdrawal symptoms are simply hangovers which are not masked by a top-up of your own particular allergen.) I can give you three examples of weekend migraine, all men as it happens, and all of whom suffered on Saturdays as a result of what happened on Fridays. The first is of a man who regularly celebrated the end of the working week by buying and consuming a single bar of chocolate. The second is of a man whose works canteen regularly served tartrazine-coloured fish for Friday lunch, and the third is of a man who 'withdrew' regularly every weekend because he was not getting the machine-dispensed-additive-laden-plastic-cup-coffee 'buzz' from consuming coffee every two to three hours at work. It all sounds very simple in *retrospect* but they all took some concentrated detective work to sort out. The answer, therefore, to discovering the cause of a weekend migraine is to ask yourself what you have been up to over the past twenty-four hours. By this means you should be able to track down the culprit.

Now we come to the problem of headaches and other symptoms associated with hypoglycaemia (low blood sugar). This can be a major problem for diabetics but migraine sufferers are not exempt. Everyone who suffers from food allergies *to any degree* is subject to hypoglycaemia. Basically it is a collection of symptoms which occur when the blood sugar level lowers through lack of food or drink. A small snack can be taken to avoid this (glucose tablets are good for those who can tolerate them as they are quickly absorbed into the blood stream – but anything else will do). Some people will find that they need to take something every two to three hours to avoid developing hypoglycaemia.

So how best can a migraine sufferer help himself? First of all, try to find out the foods and/or chemicals to which he is reacting. (After eliminating these he may well find that the triggers do not tip the balance as before.) Check on things such as whether the lenses of his glasses need changing; buy a good pair of sunglasses for the summer, take plenty of sleep, and get regular exercise in the fresh air. He should try to avoid emotional stress (easier said than done) and find time to

M

relax and make sure that he is getting all the necessary supplements. Migraine sufferers may be short of thiamine (vitamin B1) – this can be lost by consuming too much coffee – niacin (vitamin B3) and pyridoxine (vitamin B6). If self-prescribing it is better to take a strong preparation of B complex vitamins than to take these vitamins individually. Oil of Evening Primrose is helpful for all forms of allergy-induced headache, but especially for pre-menstrual headaches. Selenium is recommended for migraine sufferers and, of course, vitamin C is very important. Anyone 'working out' their allergies or in the midst of a migraine can take up to 3g a day. Once stabilised, 1g a day should be sufficient. The praises of feverfew are sung by many.

It is absolutely rotten luck being a migraine sufferer but, armed with all this information and a lot of determination, I feel sure you can beat it! Stick in there and remember: after every migraine write down what you have eaten and drunk, where you have been and what you have done in the twenty-four hours *prior* to starting your symptoms. When you have done this a few times, certain common factors should emerge. If this does not seem to throw any light on the problem, then an elimination diet with careful monitoring over the re-introduction period should provide you with the answers you are looking for.

See also **Headaches** and **Hypoglycaemia**.

MOOD SWINGS

Mood swings, ie, happy one minute and unhappy or anxious the next, if not related to circumstances can be due to food allergies, vitamin or mineral deficiencies, exposures to chemicals or hormone imbalances. Expert medical advice is needed to eliminate more serious disorders and advice on those mentioned. The problem is much simpler if the patient recognises that he suffers from mood swings. This is not always the case.

See also **Hypomania**.

MOUTH ULCERS (APHTHOUS ULCERS)

These small ulcers can appear on the tongue, inside cheek or roof of the mouth. They are painful and may last for several days. The ulcers can be caused by a minor virus infection, but if they keep recurring they are more likely to be due to an allergic reaction. People suffering from coeliac disease, Crohn's disease, migraine and ulcerative colitis are susceptible to developing mouth ulcers – as are people suffering from oral thrush and vitamin deficiencies.

Soluble aspirin in a glass of warm water swished around the mouth will help to relieve the pain, so will Mandell's paint or a dab of glycerin on the affected area.

Any food or drink or chemical additive can cause mouth ulcers. One common cause is an adverse reaction to gluten (found in wheat, oats, barley and rye), hence the connection with coeliac disease.

Malabsorption of vitamins may also play a part, so extra folic acid and vitamin B12 can be helpful. An iron supplement may also help.

MULTIPLE CHEMICAL ALLERGIES

Spare a thought for people who develop multiple chemical allergies. Their lives may become very difficult and, in some cases, may have become almost impossible. Many of them already have to contend with multiple food allergies. When their condition is very pronounced they are known as 'universal reactors'. Their GP may dismiss them because, even if he is enlightened enough to believe in multiple food allergies, he is likely to think that this is stretching credibility too far. But is it?

What have we done to our environment since the end of the last war? We have introduced into our atmosphere chemicals in the following forms: pesticides, fertilisers, insecticides, herbicides, petrochemicals, industrial air pollution, aerosols, fumes from gas, oil and petrol, exhaust fumes, formaldehyde and other industrial chemicals, and we have seriously contaminated much of our water supply. In our own homes we have actually gone out of our way to introduce chemically-based perfumes, cleaning materials, polishes, washing powders, disinfectants and air fresheners which contain formaldehyde.

We are not talking about allergies any longer but about chemical toxins, to which, in varying concentrations, nobody is immune. We all have a toxic threshold above which our body chemistry will start to break down. The universal reactors have already found themselves in this unenviable position. Sometimes they have to consider whether they will adapt their homes (often at considerable expense) or move (at even greater expense).

People can be desensitised if they can afford the treatment – many cannot – but their desensitising levels may change as they come into contact with an ever increasing number of unavoidable chemicals. Contact with other people's perfumes, smoke, exhaust fumes, etc will prohibit them from going to shops, theatres, restaurants or on public transport – anywhere in fact where they will be in contact with the human race. Some become virtually house-bound.

Superimposed on this will be a lack of understanding from most people with whom they come into contact – quite possibly including their own doctor. Theirs is a very lonely life and it would mean so much if we could spare them just a little of our time.

If you are in this category you have probably worked out already how to make your home a safe haven from the hazards of the outside world. In case you are just starting, or may have missed something (as I myself may have done on your behalf!), here are some tips. Do not allow any visitor to smoke in your home. If a member of your family smokes, ask them if they would kindly smoke outdoors if the smoke affects you. Remove all

M

polishes, bleaches, aerosols, air fresheners and strong disinfectants. Use only those cleaning materials which are absolutely essential and make sure they are not pine- or lemon-scented. Use an unscented washing up liquid and immerse the nozzle in the water before squeezing. Allow no painting or other chemical products or sprays, even in the garden. Formaldehyde affects many people. This is found in cavity wall insulation, chipboard, fabrics, disinfectants, air fresheners and in the manufacture of plastics. Get rid of plastics – they give out fumes to which you may be sensitive; the soft plastics are worse than the hard ones in this respect. The plastic components of a television set give off fumes as it heats up.

Get rid of scented toiletries – unless specifically stated they are all made from chemicals. This applies to men's toiletries, talc, after-shave and deodorants etc as well as women's – which include cosmetics, bath essence, talc, deodorants etc. Soaps, also, should be of the unscented variety. Boots the Chemist has a whole range of hypo-allergenic cosmetics which are unperfumed and, incidentally, household cleaning materials and washing products too, as do health food shops.

In the bedroom, remove as many man-made materials as you find necessary. You may be able to tolerate a polyester duvet or, if not, perhaps a feather one. As both can cause allergies you may need to resort to blankets – cotton ones if you are affected by wool. Keep the bedroom dust-free. Use a mask when dusting, and preferably a damp cloth rather than a duster. Air filters and/or an ioniser may help. If and when you do venture forth from your home try to avoid contact with factory fumes, exhaust fumes, road works, crop spraying etc. If necessary, wear a mask. do not worry about this. It is better to give everyone a laugh than feel ill! If you go out in your car and get in amongst traffic, avoid going too close to the car in front. Turn off the heater and close the air vents so as not to introduce contaminated air from outside.

It is vital to build up your strength with multi-mineral and multi-vitamin supplements which will have to be carefully suited to your individual needs. Follow the same advice as for multiple food allergy sufferers.

Your life is not easy. There are some of us around who *do* understand. We give you our support and appreciate your courage in presenting a cheerful face to the outside world in spite of the plight in which you find yourselves. I hope very much that, given time, your situation will improve.

See also **Multiple Food Allergies** and **Myalgic Encephalomyeltitis** (ME).

MULTIPLE FOOD ALLERGIES

When I kept developing more and more food allergies (in spite of discovering the cause of each one in turn) I went to my doctor in a panic and asked: 'What can I do if I become allergic to everything?'. He found this amusing and assured me there was absolutely no chance of *that*! (To give him his due it *is* unusual and I was a severe case, but not the only one.) In fact, I believe the only reason I did not continue in that vein was because I was able to make arrangements to receive enzyme-potentiated desensitisation (EPD). It is my belief that this treatment built up my immune system, thereby raising my allergy tolerance level so that the severity of my reactions was lessened and my body was better able to accept a much wider range of foods. After several months of treatment, and by avoiding those foods which caused the worst reactions, I was able to dispense with this treatment. I am convinced that this boost to my immune system coupled with the discovery that high daily doses of vitamins kept me in good health, is the reason I have stayed well ever since. This vaccine, first developed by Dr Len McEwen in 1966, has now been taken up by a number of other doctors in this country and abroad.

Of course I was not alone in this experience. Some people become allergic to a wide range of foods, making it almost impossible to find enough to give them a balanced diet (a dietician can help here). This is time-consuming, expensive and disheartening because of the difficulties in trying to find some of the more obscure foodstuffs (health food shops are your best bet). One can be tested and desensitised by another method used by some doctors: intradermal testing and desensitisation (or neutralisation). Both this and EPD will help most people but no form of treatment will suit everybody. In any case, these treatments are available only to those who can afford them or who are covered by medical insurance.

The only other alternative for multiple allergy sufferers is to rotate the foods to which they are least sensitive. To take a diet of the same limited foods every day is to lay oneself open to developing further food allergies.

On the other hand, very sensitive people who actually seem to be allergic to *all* foods are best advised to take very small amounts of a wide variety of foods (mixed together if you like) at every meal, every day. In this way, although they will never feel entirely well, they will never get a very severe reaction or suffer from lack of nutrients. I am sorry it is all so very complicated!

It is absolutely vital to build up your immune system with high doses of all the main vitamins: A, B, C, D and E, and multi-minerals too. Especially recommended are zinc, selenium, Oil of Evening Primrose and dolomite (calcium and magnesium). A firm such as Cantassium (see list of addresses) can be approached on a personal level. By making your requests for supplements known, and stating all the foods you cannot take, they will advise on what you, personally, should be able to tolerate.

See also **Multiple Chemical Allergies** and **Myalgic Encephalomyelitis** (ME).

MULTIPLE SCLEROSIS (DISSEMINATED SCLEROSIS)

Multiple sclerosis is a disease of the central nervous system in which parts of the protective covering of the nerve fibres are worn away. In Britain about one person in two thousand develops multiple sclerosis, usually around the age of thirty or so, and it is more common in women than men.

Symptoms vary from person to person, both in type and degree. Almost half of those affected start with some form of visual disturbance and/or pins and needles in the limbs. The eyes may be painful, and double vision may occur. Weakness in the limbs will cause clumsiness. A change of mood is likely, the patient becoming lighthearted or depressed or alternating between the two. He may become incontinent.

The symptoms can develop in a matter of hours or days then gradually disappear only to recur. Patients may become increasingly disabled – in some cases rapidly, but in others there will be periods of improvement (known as remission) which may last for years before another attack. A lumbar puncture test can be performed and/or visual evoked responses measured. If this confirms the presence of MS then your doctor may prescribe steroid treatment, advise rest while your symptoms are present, and arrange for a physiotherapist to give you exercises to strengthen your muscles when your symptoms abate.

MS is believed to result from a reaction to a virus. This is interesting because many people develop allergies as a result of a reaction to a virus. MS is considered to be related to a malfunctioning immune system. So are allergies. Thymosin, a natural body substance extracted from the thymus glands of cows, is used in America for people suffering from allergies, MS and other diseases to regulate the working of the immune system.

It is now known that essential fatty acids are needed for the myelination of the brain and central nervous system, and that a deficiency of these will harm them. Food processing deprives us of much of our essential fatty acids so we need to replace them in the form of cold-pressed vegetable oils. Our diet, therefore, should contain sufficient soya, corn, sunflower and safflower oils. Nuts and seeds are good too. In addition, eating fresh, fatty fish, which is very high in polyunsaturates, should help to prevent the symptoms of MS.

Doctors working in the field of allergy and environmental illness have been treating patients with MS for a number of years now. In many cases their patients have been found to respond to an elimination diet and, on the re-introduction of certain foods, their symptoms have returned. After eliminating the incriminating foods, those who have stuck religiously to their diets have remained in a state of remission or have dramatically improved.

Among the most likely causes are saturated (animal) fat, grains, particularly wheat, or the gluten in grains (found in wheat, oats, barley and rye), milk products, eggs, white sugar, chocolate, coffee, tea, alcohol and food additives (especially colourings and preservatives). Additional factors likely to be responsible are synthetic chemicals, air and water pollution.

With all this in mind, I put forward a *suggested* starting diet for MS sufferers. It may take a little while for symptoms to clear and I cannot guarantee that this diet will help everyone but it is most certainly worth trying. Once your symptoms have regressed you can re-introduce foods one at a time, monitoring as you go. However, I should strongly recommend that you *do not* return to *processed* foods with all their suspect chemical additives.

The diet I suggest is as follows. Soya, corn, sunflower and safflower oils, nuts and seeds. Any fresh fish in its natural form (avoid smoked and artificially coloured) but especially the fatty fish such as mackerel and herring. Cabbage, courgettes, leeks, carrots, celery, swede, parsnips, pears, peaches, plums, apricots, corn on the cob, brown rice, ground rice, vegetable margarine (which is free from additives) – eg, *Granose* or *Vitaquel* from health food shops. Lentils and other pulses, soya flour, maize flour, sea salt, raw cane demerara sugar, honey or fructose. Pure fruit and vegetable juices, tomato juice, soya milk, bottled water. (If your water comes from natural sources, ie, a spring or direct from chalk bore holes in the hills, then you do not need to use bottled water.) For people whose water has had to be recycled I suggest that bottled water is used for both drinking and cooking purposes. You may decide, alternatively, to investigate the advantages of a water filter.

What else is important for MS sufferers? Try to avoid sudden changes of temperature, get lots of fresh air, plenty of sleep and avoid stress as much as possible. Supplements recommended for MS sufferers are a strong multi-vitamin/multi-mineral plus extra vitamin C, 1g per day, vitamin E and vitamin A (cod liver oil is a good way to take vitamin A). Vitamins B12, B13 and folic acid are important – as are zinc, magnesium, selenium and high doses of Oil of Evening Primrose. Amino acids and digestive enzymes are thought to be beneficial also. This may sound like a great deal, but your body has reached a very low ebb and needs a lot of building up again. Inevitably there will be setbacks but you should be able to stabilise your condition by these means. If you can find a doctor specialising in allergy and environmental illness, so much the better. If you cannot (or do not have the financial means and are not covered by medical insurance) then following the above advice can do you nothing but good.

MUSCLE WEAKNESS

There are several reasons for muscle weakness, some serious, so do report it to your doctor so that he can check this out. Much is written about muscle *pain* in relation to allergies but little about muscle *weakness* – perhaps because not too many authors have been multiple allergy sufferers themselves! Muscle weakness in allergy is not unusual and is often accompanied by an overwhelming fatigue (here again your doctor should be consulted in view of all the other possible causes). Any allergic reaction can involve muscle weakness – angioedema is a common one, for example.

M

Although muscle weakness may be present in many allergic reactions, it is certainly not universal – which is what muscle-testing applied kinesiologists would have us believe. In this form of testing, the muscle strength is checked prior to a solution of an allergen being put under the tongue, after which the muscles are retested to see to what extent, if any, they have weakened. Muscle weakness is sometimes apparent, but certainly not in every reaction or for every individual. Even with soluble foods, such as sugar, there is no guarantee of an immediate reaction, and insoluble foods, such as grains, are going to take hours before they are absorbed into the blood stream. As for the alternative method, used by some practitioners, of testing the muscles before balancing a yoghurt pot on your tummy and testing again – well, that speaks for itself!

There is no documentation on foods likely to cause muscle weakness, although the glutamates 621, 622, 623 are incriminated. Also, a caffeine sensitivity, probably to coffee or tea, is possible. Milk, wheat and eggs are such common causes of allergic reaction that I would put them on the suspect list too. Coming off drugs such as corticosteroids, especially if you have been on them for a long time, often causes withdrawal symptoms such as muscle weakness, fatigue, pain and depression.

See also **Myalgic Encephalomyeltitis** (ME).

MYALGIC ENCEPHALOMYELITIS (ME/POST-VIRAL SYNDROME)

Myalgic encephalomyeltitis is an illness caused by the after-effects of 'flu or some other viral infection. It affects more than 150,000 people in Britain. This condition occurs when the immune system has over-reacted to the virus. The symptoms may include any of the following: fatigue, depression, headaches, muscle weakness, nausea, dizziness, abdominal pain, joint pains, bowel problems etc. The fatigue can be so overwhelming that the patient may easily feel incapable of making any physical or mental effort and, unfortunately, this has been construed as laziness or lack of effort by people who are ignorant of the nature of the illness.

However, a greater understanding is gradually developing, and in April 1990 the first world symposium on myalgic encephalomyelitis was held at Cambridge University. Speakers from Europe, Australia, Canada and New Zealand as well as Britain attended. All had been engaged in original research and were there to present scientific data and suggested treatments. One of the main objectives was to encourage the medical community and the Government to see this disorder as a genuine illness requiring treatment and research. Tests for ME are now available. About half of those tested show a high level of antibodies to viral proteins. If you belong to the fifty per cent whose tests were negative, do not be despondent – the tests are in their infancy; this is an illness new to the twentieth century. Lack of adequate testing does not alter the fact that if you have the symptoms you either have ME or something very like it!

M

There is no doubt that some viruses, such as glandular fever, for example, can alter our immune responses and trigger allergic reactions. ME patients are, in fact, multiple allergy sufferers who have been given a label. As such, they will benefit greatly by following an elimination diet in conjunction with the consideration of inhalant allergens. Some ME patients may have thrush also and will need treatment for this (see Candidiasis).

It must not be forgotten that a virus infection is not the only trigger. Shock, stress, hormone changes, repeated doses of drugs, exposure to chemicals and anything else which pulls a person down can lower his allergy threshold, making him susceptible to allergic reactions.

It is absolutely rotten luck to discover that you have ME, but don't give up hope. There is much that you can do to help yourself! You have become super-sensitive and you need to find out all the things you are sensitive to. Think of it as a challenge, read all you can, be a good detective and, little by little, you will find that you are making progress. Don't forget to join ME Action Campaign too (see address at back of book).

Follow advice on supplements given in the entry on **Multiple Food Allergies**.

See also **Candidiasis** and **Multiple Chemical Allergies**.

M

NASAL POLYPS

Nasal polyps are shiny nodules which grow in the nasal passages. They are caused by prolonged nasal irritation to membranes of the nose and sinuses due to allergy. They cause discomfort and a permanent feeling of congestion and can obstruct breathing. They may appear in one or both nostrils; they are not malignant but can diminish the sense of smell and taste.

Nasal polyps are usually accompanied by rhinitis (sneezing and runny, itchy nose). They will persist if untreated. They can be removed by surgery but are likely to recur if the cause is not identified.

The only recorded causes are wheat, food additives (namely azo dyes, benzoate preservatives and metabisulphites) and a sensitivity to salicylates. The latter are found in aspirin (there are many over-the-counter preparations which contain aspirin). Paracetamol does not contain aspirin and can be used without ill effect by most allergy sufferers. Remember that anything which causes constant irritation to your nasal passages (ie symptoms of hay fever) can be a cause, or increase your chances of developing nasal polyps. Even a nasal spray, if you over use it, can irritate the nasal passages and cause polyps.

Vitamin C is a natural antihistamine. One gramme taken three times a day has proved successful in getting rid of nasal polyps in some cases but this dose should be decreased to 1g a day after a few weeks whether or not the nasal polyps disappear.

See also **Hay Fever** and **Smell and Taste, Lack of Sense of**.

NAUSEA

Nausea is a very common symptom for which there are many causes. It may on occasions be accompanied by diarrhoea. Among the more common causes are gastritis, gastroenteritis (food poisoning), over-eating or drinking too much alcohol, travel sickness, caffeine sensitivity, migraine and other allergic reactions. Pregnant women are prone to feeling nauseous especially in the early morning during the first three months. (A dry biscuit and a warm drink when you wake up can do wonders.) They may find certain foods or drinks such as tea and coffee nauseous throughout the whole of their pregnancy. (In any case they would be better off without them.)

Among the more likely causes of a feeling of nausea in food intolerance are milk, wheat, eggs and the caffeine-containing products – coffee, tea, chocolate and cola.

Feeling nauseous is a common reaction to inhaled chemicals when the patient may feel faint or dizzy also. Nausea is experienced by many people, especially youngsters, when travelling by car. They may be reacting to the fumes of the interior of a new car or, alternatively, other people's

N

exhaust fumes coming in through the air vents or windows. Earl Mindell, in *The Vitamin Bible*, recommends 100mg of a preparation of B complex vitamins to be taken before a journey in order to prevent travel sickness. B1 (thiamine) and B6 (pyridoxine) are said to be effective in relieving nausea, but if self-prescribing it is probably better to take them in the form of a B complex preparation.

See also **Travel Sickness**.

NECK PAIN

If stiffness or pain in the neck is accompanied by a severe headache, fever or vomiting, you should contact your doctor immediately. Stiffness of the neck may occur following an injury or trauma such as a car accident. It can also be caused by draughts; some people are particularly susceptible this way.

However, a stiff neck may start suddenly for no apparent reason and it can be very painful on moving. It may be diagnosed as fibrositis, which is pain in the shoulder and neck muscles. Although the cause is not known, damp conditions bring it on in some people. With rest and patience it usually clears up within a few days. If it goes on for longer than a week, consult your doctor.

Stiffness and pain in the neck, possibly with face or shoulder pain as well, can most certainly be the result of an allergy to a food and maybe to an inhaled chemical as well. (It is a not uncommon symptom of withdrawal when on an elimination diet, especially for those suffering from arthritis.) Suspect foods are coffee, tea, milk, wheat, corn, cheese, yeast, chocolate, citrus fruits, sugar, pork, food additives especially colourings, monosodium glutamate and sodium nitrite.

See also **Aches and Pains**, **Arthritis**, and **Shoulder, Stiffness in**.

N

NERVOUS BREAKDOWN

The term 'nervous breakdown' has no precise medical meaning. We use it to describe the condition of someone who, for one reason or another, becomes unable to carry on his job and/or family responsibilities. This breakdown can take any form, producing either physical or mental symptoms, usually both. In the majority of cases no one is to blame. Everyone has a breaking point, given the necessary circumstances. There should be no stigma, rather compassion and understanding and a realisation that 'there but for the grace of God' go the rest of us.

People suffering from a nervous breakdown will initially need a good listener, if they are able to unburden themselves. The listener will need to be just that, even if he thinks the worries are quite unjustified. Later one, when the patient is over the critical period, it may be possible to explain gently that he may have had things out of perspective.

With regard to treatment, some methods work for some, others for another. Some drugs, as a temporary measure, can be very effective – indeed, may be necessary until the patient can be stabilised. Other people may benefit from psychotherapy, especially those people who feel inferior or inadequate. So what if you are not as clever/beautiful/talented as the next person? You can be kind/helpful/conscientious and which, in the end, is the most important? Everyone has their worth, yes *everybody*, and you are no exception. If you *want* to get better, you *will* get better. In the end it comes down to you.

One can fight anything if one wants to. A breakdown happens either through unfortunate circumstances or poor health, but frequently both. A thorough medical check-up is essential, as a physical cause – such as a hormone imbalance – may be part of the problem. Once the physical side has been dealt with, the circumstances surrounding the breakdown must be considered. If you cannot change your circumstances, then you have to change your attitude. If, by putting up a fight, you *can* change your circumstances, then you have to decide whether, given time, you are prepared to do this. You can do much to help yourself with the incredible healing power of positive thought. Do not allow negative thoughts to enter your mind. If they do: banish them. If we can brainwash ourselves into becoming ill we can certainly brainwash ourselves back to good health.

I once read a moving story in the *Reader's Digest* of a man who was hospitalised as a result of a breakdown due to the very stressful circumstances of his life. He lay in bed, sick and weak and unresponsive to treatment, and the doctors had to admit they were baffled. The man reasoned that if a combination of sad and distressing circumstances had caused his illness, was it not logical to assume that happy, joyful circumstances would reverse the situation? I forget the exact details, but I do remember that he was prescribed his favourite music and the television and radio programmes which made him laugh the most, and this resulted in the turning point of his illness – after which he made a good and sound recovery. Life is not always so simple.

You are probably wondering what any of this has to do with allergies and environmental illness. Well, it hasn't, but it has to be mentioned first! If you can now say 'yes, I know all this, I want to get better, I have put all you say into practice but I feel worse than ever', then I say to you: 'Perhaps you are suffering from sensitivities to foods or chemicals which you have not even considered.'

When I was (unwittingly) developing a caffeine sensitivity (in spite of the fact that I was usually a one-cup-a-day girl), I reached the point where my body decided enough was enough and I had a very severe and frightening adverse reaction. When the doctor arrived he diagnosed 'stress', patted me on the hand and left. One tends to define the word stress as circumstantial, and I knew this could not be the case as I had no particular worries at that time.

However, what I did not know then – but learned later – was that caffeine could have an effect on the central nervous system causing all sorts of emotional symptoms such as anxiety, nervousness, fear, shaking, depression, loss of confidence and acute fatigue. This fact is now better understood, caffeine being recognised as a drug and a stimulant. What is not so well documented is that even a very small amount can affect sensitised people and that, in fact, *any* food or drink can affect the central nervous system in the same manner. This is not necessarily because of what it contains but because of the response of the body chemistry of the individual.

Therefore, to have any chance of coping with the hazards of everyday living one needs to be on top of one's allergies. The symptoms which cause someone to feel they cannot cope can be caused not only by caffeine-containing products but also by foods such as milk, wheat, eggs etc. Drugs, food additives and chemical inhalants, smoking and drinking may all have the same effect. Hormone imbalances should be investigated, too, by an endocrinologist, if necessary.

You have been, or are going, through a terrible time. No one knows the extent to which you have suffered. Discover and recognise the causes which have contributed, whatever they may be, and you *will* recover. It will take time but every day you are one step nearer. A strong preparation of B complex vitamins can work wonders.

See also **Mental Illness**.

NERVOUSNESS

Nervousness is usually accompanied by other symptoms such as anxiety, fear, lack of confidence, depression, acute fatigue and so on, but it may simply be present on its own. If you feel nervous of everyday situations and shy away from human contact you probably think of this as your own personality. Of course you may be right, but equally it may be the effects of caffeine, other foods or drinks, chemical inhalants, alcohol, smoking or even the side-effects of any drugs you may be taking.

For years I was a smoker because I believed that I needed cigarettes to calm my 'nerves'. It was only after I gave up smoking that I realised that it was the cigarettes which had caused my nervousness!

There is a recognised allergic condition called the tension–fatigue syndrome in which the patient's brain won't stop rushing around in circles and therefore leaves him constantly exhausted. This is enough to put anyone into a nervous state. Try to find the cause by eliminating the offending items and life will become much more comfortable.

See also **Mental Illness**, **Nervous Breakdown** and **Tension/Fatigue Syndrome**.

NIGHTMARES

Much nonsense, I believe, is written about dreams. Of *course* it is

N

fun to fantasise and imagine all sort of weird and wonderful reasons and interpretations for what we dream – so long as we can separate fantasy from fact.

I suggest that we dream for one of two reasons and, more often than not, as the result of a combination of both. Either our dreams are related in some way to our hopes or worries, or they are just related to events in our lives regarding our own circumstances, or those of someone close to us. (Occasionally some odd-bod pops up at random for no apparent reason!) Anyone who has any personal worries is much more likely to dream than someone who is content with his lot in life. When these dreams are particularly frightening or traumatic we call them nightmares.

The other reason we dream is because we have stimulated our brains with the effects of caffeine, alcohol, foods, food additives, spices, chemical inhalants or drugs. Some of us have brains which require very little stimulation! Such people can suffer the most horrendous nightmares which can be just as terrifying as anything which happens in real life. Children who suffer from nightmares need much comforting and understanding.

Taking a strong preparation of B complex vitamins does help to calm down the nervous system, and the avoidance last thing at night of foods like cheese, which are known to be indigestible, will help – but you *do* need to discover the causes. From personal experience I find the caffeine-containing drinks and certain spices the worst. Drugs are very dicey as they are likely to contain colourings, preservatives and flavourings, and some contain caffeine as well.

See also **Insomnia**.

NIPPLES, ITCHING

There are a number of breast problems which can arise for lactating women which are not covered here. For everyone else, changes in the nipples are rare, but if the skin should start to pucker or change colour, or a discharge be noted, then you should consult your doctor without delay.

The nipples, being a sensitive area, are sometimes prone to eczema. This will cause itching. It may be a weeping eczema which quickly hardens and forms a crust covering the nipple. One or both nipples may be affected. The most likely cause will be a food or drink. Milk, milk products, eggs or pork are the most suspect. It is also possible that the material from which your bra is made – or even the thread with which it is stiched could be a source of irritation causing contact eczema.

See also **Eczema**.

OBESITY

Being overweight is detrimental to health and makes people more susceptible to certain other diseases. For one thing, it imposes extra strain on the heart. A small number of cases of obesity are related to medical conditions, such as hormonal imbalance. So, if in doubt (or other symptoms are present) do go to your doctor for a check-up. People tend to put on weight due to hormonal changes, during the 'change of life' for example, but this is quite normal.

For the most part it is just that some people burn up their food at a slower rate than others so have to eat less to maintain a reasonable weight. This seems very unfair – considering that most of us enjoy our food and think of it as one of Life's pleasures. Life *is* unfair, though, so there is no point in dwelling on it!

Sugary and starchy foods are the ones which make us put on weight. These are sweets, cake, chocolate, pastries, jam, bread and potatoes, and some snacks. Excessive dieting can be dangerous, and is also quite pointless because most people will give it up after a short while and regain their lost weight. It is far better to diet in moderation and try to replace the fattening foods with more fruit and vegetables; that is a far healthier diet, anyway. Try to avoid processed foods which usually contain hidden sugar, and I advise cutting out canned drinks and squashes altogether and replacing them with natural fruit or vegetable juices. Cutting down on sugar is important, and replacing it (where this is essential) with honey or fructose is better.

When people are compulsive eaters, this is usually either psychological (because they are compensating for their dissatisfaction with life) or it is the result of an allergy. These may in fact be interrelated more often than is realised. Overweight through overeating usually means addiction, and the most common foods to which people get addicted are coffee, tea, chocolate, wheat, corn, sugar and alcohol. (An addiction to alcohol is often to one of its constituents rather than to the alcohol itself.)

To overcome an addiction you have to face up to it and accept that in giving it up you are likely to suffer withdrawal symptoms initially. The best way to get over the craving of an addiction is to eliminate the food or drink in question. Take 1g of vitamin C three times a day, take one teaspoonful of sodium bicarbonate in a glass of warm water three times a day, and get out into the fresh air as often as possible. Take plenty of fresh fruit and vegetables, meat, fish or pulses, and drink plenty of water. When you are over the *worst* of the withdrawal symptoms (which should be within a week) cut down the vitamin C to 1g a day and cut out the sodium bicarbonate altogether.

One strange phenomenon – but a common problem for food-allergy sufferers – is the ability to put on weight quite disproportionately to the amount of food taken. There are case histories of the woman who puts

O

on four pounds after eating a spoonful of cottage cheese, and the man who adds seven pounds after taking a single peanut. The reason for this is that allergic people can add five to twenty-five pounds in oedema (fluid retention) at a sitting! Certain foods, therefore, in some people, cause swelling to such a degree that they find it necessary to own different sizes of clothing to fit their different requirements. They feel and look as if they are pregnant – men too!

The oedema experienced by many women prior to menstruating can be related to foods which are affecting them at a time when they are more than usually susceptible.

Salt is known to cause water retention so, for people prone to oedema, a salt-free diet is recommended. Other foods most commonly incriminated are wheat, corn, milk, eggs, sugar and peanuts.

Iodine is known to burn off excess fat. One of the best ways in which to take it is in the form of kelp, a supplement made from seaweed, which also contains other excellent properties. (Anyone taking replacement thyroid should do this only under medical supervision as kelp affects the thyroid gland.)

For everyone trying to slim, therefore, whatever the basic cause, try to take a diet free from salt and sugary and starchy foods, drink lots of water, take as much *gentle* exercise as you can, and don't forget the kelp!

See also **Addiction** and **Bulimia**.

OFFICE BUILDING SYNDROME (SICK BUILDING SYNDROME)

It is not uncommon for people to develop symptoms which are related to their place of work. One of the major reasons for the 'office building syndrome' is the use of air conditioners. These can cause micro-organisms to grow. They also harbour certain moulds, especially during the winter months; when circulated, these moulds can cause allergic reactions. Some air conditioners are run by gas or oil (two other common allergens). Some bring in air from outside including tree, grass and flower pollens when in season.

Inside the office there are fumes from photocopiers, Tipp-Ex, print and so on to which some people will be sensitive. People who are constantly exposed to chemicals as a result of their jobs may easily become sensitised to them and develop symptoms as a result. Typical examples are hairdressers, dry cleaners, office cleaners and those who work in pharmaceutical companies. If you suspect your workplace of being responsible for your symptoms then taking a few days off, perhaps over a holiday period, will clarify whether or not this is the cause of your problems. You may suffer withdrawal symptoms initially for a few days, after which you should begin to feel much better. If the symptoms reappear after you return to work this would seem to prove the point.

PALATE, ITCHING

The only reference I can find to this symptom is in Dr Paul Carson's book *How to Cope with your Child's Allergies*, in which he says under the heading of 'Hay fever': 'Occasionally there is an intense itch along the roof of the mouth and inside the ears.' This is a very persistent symptom which may come with other hay fever symptoms or it may be present on its own.

The most common causes are pollens, animal dander or chemicals, especially perfumes or scented cleaning materials. Less frequently it is caused by foods or food additives.

See also **Hay Fever**.

PALLOR

Pallor usually indicates poor health. There are exceptions. A few people are naturally pale though perfectly well. Others always look red-cheeked and robust, even when ill. In the majority of cases a sick person looks sick, and those who suffer from allergies particularly so. Children usually have dark, puffy circles under their eyes (known as 'allergic shiners'), look tired, may have a blocked up nose, are nervous and are invariably pale. They may be drowsy, listless, confused, depressed, emotional (or apathetic), irritable and have poor co-ordination. On the other hand, they may be restless, awkward, clumsy, disruptive, excitable and quite unable to keep still, depending on which way their allergies affect them.

Adults can have the same problems but they are not always so easily categorised. Anyone, child or adult, who is under par, and for whom no satisfactory medical explanation has yet been given, may well be either eating the wrong diet or suffering from undetected allergies.

See also **General Feeling of Being Unwell** and **Zombie-like State**.

P

PALPITATIONS

In the normal run of things we are unaware of our heart beating, although it certainly makes itself felt in times of stress. There is a world of difference between the speeded up action of the heart-beat due to a change in our emotions and the extraordinary sensation of palpitations.

This can be a frightening experience, and people should always be checked by their doctors in case it is related to a recognised heart disorder. Quite often, however, this is found not to be the case, and no cause can be given. However, palpitations can be caused by an adverse reaction to things such as tea, coffee, alcohol or smoking, even when these have appeared to cause no problem in the past.

Palpitations can be so severe as to make a person believe he is dying. In fact, distressing though this is, when related to an allergic reaction, it is not in itself in any way dangerous. The most common causes are caffeine-containing products – tea, coffee, chocolate, cola drinks or caffeine-containing over-the-counter drugs. Milk, wheat and eggs have been implicated, but other foods and drinks may also be responsible. Chemical additives have a lot to answer for. Particularly suspect are the glutamates 621, 622, 623.

See also **Heart Conditions.**

PANIC ATTACKS

It is only too easy to observe someone in a panic and have the attitude that they are over-reacting, especially if there appears to be no specific reason for panicking.

Doctors who work in the field of allergy and environmental illness are aware that foods, food additives, natural or chemical inhalants, stings or injections can provoke reactions which can cause anaphylactic shock and death. That is allergy in its severest form and is relatively rare. Nevertheless, there are degrees of severity. As an onlooker, never underestimate the need to take an allergic reaction seriously. In some cases it is obvious when the patient is in distress, in others it is not. The complexities of the immune response are not yet fully understood. Suffice to say that some people are capable of producing severe reactions in certain circumstances. The onset of the symptoms may be almost immediate, or they may come on extraordinarily suddenly even after a delay of several hours. An experience of this nature can be terrifying and traumatic, and the patient often feels he is about to die (although in fact he is not). Naturally, he panics. To this patient I say the following: 'You are not going to die. You are going to be alright. Lie down on your bed or the sofa – or on the floor if need be. Be still, try to keep calm. You *are* going to be alright. You are very frightened. I know. I understand. Try to relax. It will pass. Give it time and it will pass. Just relax. In time you may be able to sleep a little. You will feel better when you wake up.' See also **Claustrophobia.**

PEPTIC ULCER

A peptic ulcer can mean a gastric (stomach) ulcer or a duodenal ulcer. When a part of the lining of the stomach or duodenum is eroded by the effects of the digestive juices an ulcer will form, causing pain and inflammation. Antacids are recommended in order to neutralise the hydrochloric acid formed in the stomach. These will give the ulcer a chance to heal and are used in conjunction with other drugs.

Symptoms are a pain in the stomach after meals, probably accompanied by excessive wind and possibly a feeling of nausea. These symptoms can also occur at other times and can be relieved by eating or by taking further medication. Contributory factors are considered to be smoking, too much alcohol, too many fried foods, the effects of aspirin and other drugs and/or a rushed, stressed life style. Peptic ulcers require medical attention.

It is also possible to suffer from peptic-ulcer-type pain without positive X-ray evidence of an ulcer, in which case the pain is likely to be allergic in origin.

In orthodox treatment, a bland diet is recommended and this usually means milk in order to counteract the effect of too much acid production. This is fine unless it turns out to be the very food which is causing the symptoms – in which case the patient will become a good deal worse. Pain relieved by drinking milk in the middle of the night is likely to be a masked allergy (see Elimination Diet, Chapter 5). There have been several case histories where foods have been incriminated, and the most common ones have turned out to be milk, sugar, white flour, spiced and pickled foods. Certain additives have been found to be responsible for causing ulcers; these are: E220, E230, E232, E241, 620, 621, 622, 623, Quillaia (Quillaja) – used as a foaming agent and a flavouring, and xylitol, used as a sweetening agent and a humectant (to keep foods moist).

Recommended supplements are vitamin A, vitamin C – 1g daily, a strong preparation of B complex vitamins, and a good multi-mineral. Alfalfa (from health food shops) is said to be good too. Cabbage juice has also been found to be beneficial in treating peptic ulcers.

PHOTOTOXICITY (PHOTOSENSITIVITY)

Phototoxicity (photosensitivity) refers to a condition where the skin becomes extra sensitive to sunlight. People affected may develop 'sun-burn' or come out in a rash after a short exposure to sunlight (or, in severe cases, just to daylight). This can happen even when the outside temperature is too low to affect anyone else. It may be the result of a rare medical disorder or a vitamin deficiency but these are both very unlikely and by far the most common causes are the side-effects of certain drugs. The only satisfactory answer is to give up taking the particular drug concerned, but this must be done only in consultation with your doctor – who may wish to prescribe another in its place. Photosensitivity can also be caused by the Pill, antidepressants or tranquillisers – or even by antihistamines. Photosensitivity is the result of chemicals within the body reacting to sunlight. It can also occur from chemical changes due to pregnancy but then it will right itself after your baby is born. Certain chemical food additives have also been incriminated, especially the colour erythrosine (E127) found in certain brands of glacé cherries.

Phototoxicity is not to be confused with photophobia, which is the sensitivity of the eyes to bright light or sunshine as experienced some-times, for example, by migraine sufferers.

In *The Vitamin Bible* Earl Mindell says that 'skin that is particularly sensitive to sunlight is often an early indication of niacin deficiency.' (Niacin, also known as nicotinic acid, niacinamide or nicotinamide, is

P

vitamin B3.) Mindell also tells us that niacin on its own should be used cautiously by anyone with severe diabetes, glaucoma, peptic ulcers or impaired liver function.

PILL, ADVERSE EFFECTS OF

The Pill, known also as oral contraception, was introduced in the 1960s. With it many women saw themselves as being 'liberated'. In fact, those who used it brought upon themselves a whole host of problems.

Oral contraceptives are steroids. As such they can cause serious hormonal side-effects. Dr Ellen Grant (author of *The Bitter Pill*), who worked at London's Charing Cross Hospital, has done in-depth studies on the Pill and is most concerned about the common practise of prescribing pill hormones to teenagers for period problems or contraception. Young women are especially likely to develop serious chemical imbalances leading to multiple allergies and long-term reproduction difficulties.

Steroids suppress the immune system. This encourages allergies and the growth of intestinal thrush (which in itself can lead to further allergies). Women who are on the Pill and who smoke further increase their chances of developing food allergies. Migraine is the most common manifestation of allergic illness induced by the Pill but allergy can take many forms. It has been proved that many women who give up the Pill subsequently lose their migraine and other allergies. Taking the Pill encourages more allergies, infections and auto-immune disease but this fact is kept well hidden because of the inconvenience of public concern.

Women who develop food allergies as a result of taking the Pill may find that they have become sensitive to everyday foods such as wheat, milk or eggs, but any food may be involved – as indeed, may chemical inhalants. The Pill also alters the nutritional balance, so women may become short of zinc, magnesium, manganese or iron. A strong multi-mineral supplement, therefore, is advisable, together with a strong preparation of B complex vitamins to redress the balance.

PINS AND NEEDLES (TINGLING)

This is a sensation we have all experienced at one time or another. Pressure on a nerve causes the limb to 'go to sleep'. Moving position will make it go away.

When 'pins and needles' cannot be made to disappear at will, it may be due to a number of causes – neuritis (inflammation of a nerve) for one. It is true that this is a symptom of multiple sclerosis, but as only one person in two thousand develops it in Britain the chances are remote. However, should this symptom continue, and if other symptoms are present, you would be well advised to consult your doctor. If he declares that he can find nothing wrong, then it is probably an allergy-induced symptom of the nervous system.

P

'Pins and needles' can be caused by anything, but the most likely culprits are coffee, tea, chocolate, cola, milk, wheat, eggs, sugar and pork.

PREGNANCY (ADVICE ON)

So many more babies are being born predisposed to allergy (or have already been sensitised in the womb) that it is more essential than it has ever been for prospective mothers to have the knowledge of the best means of avoiding this.

To give a baby his very best chance of good health, ideally *both* parents should avoid such hazards as alcohol, smoking and drugs (street, medical or self-prescribed) for at least three months before the intended conception. After conception, the mother-to-be should spend her pregnancy in the healthiest possible environment, eating a varied diet of pure foods. As the first fifty-six days of conception are the most important, this means starting as soon as you *hope* you have conceived rather than waiting until after it has been confirmed. Babies born between September and February are less likely to develop pollen-related hay fever.

A major hormone change takes place after a woman conceives, and there is a definite connection between hormones and allergies. Some women say that pregnancy makes them feel 'on top of the world' and others feel considerably less well than usual, sometimes very nauseous. Early morning sickness for the first three months is not abnormal as the body adapts to its hormonal changes (a warm drink and a dry biscuit when you wake will help considerably) but prolonged severe vomiting is abnormal. The greatly increased sense of smell which some women experience may be related to developing inhalant sensitivities which, in turn, cause the vomiting. Discovering and avoiding these can eliminate the need for drugs.

As it is now known that it is possible to sensitise a baby before it is born, it is essential that a prospective mother avoid all her known allergens plus anything (food or inhalant) which makes her feel ill whilst pregnant. She must eat a healthy, balanced diet (if in doubt consult a dietitian) not overdoing any specific food. Milk, wheat and eggs, being the most common allergens, should be limited. It is a mistake to drink large quantities of milk. Cut down drastically on caffeine and alcohol. Erik Millstone, in *Additives – a Guide for Everyone*, says: 'The human foetus is potentially vulnerable to caffeine and so in 1980 the Commissioner of the US Food and Drug Administration advised pregnant women to restrict and diminish their caffeine intake.' Some authorities recommend giving them up altogether as they are said to prevent a child reaching his full potential. Try to drink lots of water and fruit (or vegetable) juices instead.

Smoking increases the risk of a baby developing allergies, so it is important to cut this out. Luckily, many pregnant women do not feel like smoking anyway. As putting on too much weight is an added risk factor, 'eat little and often' would seem to be a good maxim. Avoid all chemical

P

additives. The fewer processed foods you have the better. Watch out for carrageenan (E407) which is suspected of possibly having a toxic effect on embryos. If any drugs have to be prescribed, check with your doctor that these are safe to take during pregnancy (your chemist can confirm this for you or advise on the best alternative). Watch out for becoming anaemic – a common condition in pregnant women. If it should become necessary for you to take iron, ask to have it prescribed in the form of *Sytron* which is iron in its natural form, free from artificial colouring and other additives.

All the advice on diet applies equally to a mother who is breast-feeding – as a baby can be sensitised via her milk. Drinking a lot of milk is definitely not recommended – fruit juices and water are preferable. Nevertheless, there are many benefits to your baby in breast-feeding him for as long as possible. If you should find you are having difficulty in producing breast milk, it may be that you have an undetected allergy to cow's milk and, once this is eliminated from your diet, your breast-milk should flow in. If your baby is to be born in hospital, make sure that the staff are aware that you want to breast-feed from the start. It is important not to take the Pill whilst breast-feeding.

Earl Mindell, in *The Vitamin Bible*, recommends the following supplements for pregnant women. 'A good, high potency multiple vitamin and mineral rich in vitamins A, B6, B12, C and folic acid. Multiple chelated minerals, rich in calcium (2 tablets should equal 1000mg calcium and 500mg magnesium). One of each twice daily. Also, folic acid, 800mcg three times a day. Nursing mothers need the same plus additional vitamins A, B6, B12 and C. Your body and your baby need the best nourishment you can give them.'

If you should come across this advice too late, or if you are not in a position to follow it to the letter, *do not worry*. Most pregnant mums have never read a thing and they produce bonny, bouncing babies.

PRE-MENSTRUAL SYNDROME (PMS)

This condition, from which about forty per cent of women are believed to suffer, is sometimes known as pre-menstrual tension (PMT). However, pre-menstrual syndrome is a better description as so many symptoms other than tension can be involved. These include mood swings, depression, fatigue, headache, oedema (bloating caused by water retention), breast tenderness, abdominal pain, backache, irritability, tearfulness, insomnia and in severe cases, rages and near suicidal depression. Naturally, these can have a disastrous effect on work capabilities and personal relationships.

The symptoms (and not every one suffers from all of them, thank goodness) can start from two to ten days before a menstrual period and usually last from two to seven days. They are caused by changes in the hormonal balance which can lead to a build-up of fluids in the body.

P

Diuretic tablets to eliminate the oedema may help. Some women with severe symptoms may be lacking in the hormone progesterone and can be treated for this.

Poor nutrition contributes to both physical and mental stress and much can be done for women suffering from pre-menstrual symptoms by correcting their diets. Many of them are eating unbalanced diets. It will help enormously if you can cut out smoking, alcohol, coffee, tea, chocolate, white sugar and salt altogther. Also, cut out junk foods, ie, processed foods with chemical additives. This is easier said than done, I know, but they are likely to be contributing greatly to your problems. Try to stick to a diet of pure foods with plenty of fresh fruit and vegetables.

Many doctors have found that a number of their pre-menstrual patients have much improved after going on to an elimination diet (see Chapter 5) but this may not be necessary for everyone if they follow the advice already given. The start of an elimination diet, in these circumstances, should be planned to start five days or more before you would expect your pre-menstrual symptoms to start and continue until after you would expect them to finish. If they do not appear, or are much subdued, then you know you are on the right track.

Foods attributed to causing pre-menstrual symptoms (in addition to those mentioned before) include milk, eggs, cheese, citrus fruits, wheat and red wine. Certain common inhalant allergens such as car exhaust fumes, perfumes, pollution etc, may play a part also. Try to avoid anything suspect, particularly at that time. In many cases both food and inhalant allergens may need to be avoided only during the time when you would normally suffer from pre-menstrual symptoms.

Some women have this problem as a result of thrush. When the thrush is treated, the symptoms clear up. Plenty of fresh air and exercise are an essential part of keeping fit. Vitamin and mineral supplements are required to correct abnormal hormone levels. Taking the following will help: a strong preparation of multi-vitamin/multi-mineral, Vitamin B6, magnesium, calcium, vitamin E and Oil of Evening Primrose. Products containing a proper balance of all these supplements can now be bought in health food shops. They go under names like *Lady Care*.

If your pre-menstrual tension is too much for you to handle, even after you have taken all the above advice, then you can contact the Premenstrual Tension Advisory Service (see address page 204).

P

PRURITIS (ALSO SPELT PRURITUS)

Pruritis means itching. Pruritis ani is itching around the anus, with or without a rash, and it can affect both men and women. Men can also suffer from itching or rashes on the penis. Pruritis vulvae is inflammation and itching of the skin surrounding the entrance to the vagina. This type of itching can be very intense and distressing and can keep the sufferer awake at night.

Pruritis is a common symptom in diabetes and jaundice and, if your doctor suspects either of these, they can be tested for through blood and urine samples. Itching can be due to thrush in either men or women and, if necessary, your doctor can take a swab to confirm this.

In the majority of cases the itching is due to allergy. This can be an allergy to a detergent or fabric conditioner or underwear made from a synthetic material, or any scented toiletries. For women, also, it may be due to a reaction to a tampon or contraceptive. In most cases, however, and where other complaints have been ruled out, itching of the vagina, penis or anus will be due to an allergy to a food or drink. This could be to one of many things, but suspect first anything which has been chemically processed such as tea (herb teas also), coffee, and processed foods containing artificial additives; particularly suspect are Indigo Carmine E132, black pepper and other spices.

Scratching is almost unavoidable because the itch is so intense. Just make sure that you have washed your hands otherwise you could add infection to your problems. Take frequent baths and add a cup of cooking salt to your bath water. Your doctor can prescribe an antihistamine to relieve the itching and/or a steroid cream, and this will be helpful as a temporary measure. TCP ointment is excellent for removing the itch but expect it to sting initially; it is very strong and should be used with caution. All these tips will help to relieve the situation; however, they are not going to cure the condition, so it is necessary to look for the cause.

Recommended supplements are a strong preparation of B complex vitamins and acidophilus culture.

PSORIASIS

Psoriasis is a non-infectious scaly eruption of the skin. It tends to begin in childhood or early adulthood. The onset in children can be sudden. Spots develop in stages and merge together to form deep red, scaly patches the centre of which may revert to normal – leaving circular patches. It usually affects the skin near the joints – such as inside the elbows or behind the knees – although other areas are often involved too. The scalp is sometimes affected, but not the face. Attacks may start following an infection, stress or the taking of drugs. The patches commonly heal in due course, only to recur. Doctors may prescribe various treatments, including steroid creams which can be helpful on a temporary basis.

A number of doctors working in the field of environmental illness believe this condition to be caused by a food allergy, and those foods most commonly implicated are milk, wheat, cheese, eggs, citrus fruits and a variety of food additives. As some skin conditions can be caused by inhalant allergens (though rarely) this is always another possibility.

However, Dr John Mansfield believes psoriasis to be linked with candidiasis (thrush), and he refers to psoriatic arthritis (meaning the condition where psoriasis is accompanied by arthritis) in his book *Ar-*

thritis – the Allergy Connection. He quotes Professor Rosenberg of Memphis, USA, as saying that psoriasis is an inherited fault in the body's antigen/antibody response to foreign organisms, especially *Candida albicans*. Dr Mansfield has found with his own patients that, in the majority of cases of psoriatic arthritis, the arthritis is due to food allergy but the psoriasis is due to *Candida*. In a smaller number of cases, he says, the psoriasis *and* the arthritis have responded to candida treatment. Not all doctors agree with Dr Mansfield, and some have not found psoriasis to be linked with *Candida*; instead, they have found that it responds to the food allergy approach.

PULSE RATE, ABNORMAL

A normal pulse rate ranges between fifty-five and eighty-five beats a minute, depending on age and circumstances – seventy beats a minute being about average obviously rising after exercise. A racing pulse (or slower than normal pulse) denotes a change in the body chemistry.

In the 1950s Dr Arthur Coca declared that an allergic reaction could cause an increase in the heart-beat and pulse. He devised a test involving checking the pulse both before and after consuming a suspect food and continuing to take it at regular intervals to note whether there had been a change. (An alternative to eating the food is to dilute it and put it under the tongue because this will produce a quicker result. This is known as sublingual testing.)

To check your pulse you place your index finger and second fingers on the artery on the inside of your wrist. This test is based on the belief that allergic reactions cause the release of adrenalin. Undoubtedly they do in many reactions, but not necessarily in all. Even when this does happen, there will be varying delays with different foods, even in the same person.

In addition, the pulse changes with any psychological or emotional stress, and many other factors could easily intervene. For these and further reasons which might cause both false-positives and false-negatives, this test has become more or less obsolete. In any case, why, one might ask, is it necessary to test for a reaction of which one is all too aware? This is because the rise in pulse is often a precursor to other symptoms which will follow.

P

RAPIDLY CHANGING SYMPTOMS

For the time being there is no simple satisfactory test which can conclusively prove that someone is susceptible to allergies or intolerances. There are some tests which prove some symptoms in some instances with some people, and there are tests for each individual allergen, but that is all. For this reason, sceptical doctors have been able to get away with their scepticism, and many a patient, who may understand far more about the subject than the doctor, has been discouraged by his attitude.

If you have been to your doctor (and maybe others), if you have seen specialists, if you have been for hospital tests and nothing has come to light, do consider allergies. Do not allow yourself to be brain-washed into believing that your problems are psychological before considering this as a strong possibility. Remember – there are many bogus 'experts' who are advertising allergy testing and whose methods are totally non-scientific. Go only to a qualified doctor, preferably one whose name has been given by an allergy association.

If your symptoms change frequently, so that you may be ill one day and better the next, or better and worse within a few hours or even minutes, this typifies allergy. It can be quite frightening – the speed at which allergic reactions appear and, just when you are resigned to being ill, you are feeling better! The symptoms can, of course, be constant where someone is in regular contact with an allergen. However, rapidly fluctuating symptoms which may bear no apparent relationship to one another are very indicative of allergy.

RASHES, SKIN

A rash is the name for an eruption of the skin. Rashes come in many forms and for different reasons. It is the body's reaction to some form of irritation which can be either physical or allergic in origin. Rashes which appear with infectious diseases are likely to affect the whole body and will probably be accompanied by fever and other symptoms. I refer to the childhood diseases of measles, German measles, chicken pox and so on.

Rashes without other symptoms can be due to a number of causes of which allergy or some form of sensitivity is a common one. Some are itchy, some are not, and they may come and go or simply persist until the reason for them is found and eradicated.

Nalcrom (sodium cromoglycate) is an effective allergy blocker for rashes caused by food allergy but it is not advisable to take it all the time. Antihistamine creams and ointments are sometimes very effective in clearing up skin rashes but, again, these should be used only as a temporary measure. (A few people may even produce an allergic reaction to their antihistamine cream.)

There is a wide variety of possible causes for allergic rashes and I

R

do not profess to have included them all. They can be caused by food allergy, inhalant allergy or contact allergy. The most usual foods are milk, wheat, eggs, cheese, citrus fruits, coffee, tea, chocolate, cola, food additives, especially azo and coal-tar dyes such as tartrazine. A very common cause is the effects of a drug (or one of the colourings or other chemicals added to the drug). Inhalant allergens include gas, smoke, perfumes, paint etc. Contactants include perfumes, toiletries, nickel, household cleaning materials, detergents, chemical irritants, clothing made from synthetic materials, woollens, typewriter ink and other office materials, cosmetics, pharmaceutical creams and lanolin. Some rashes are due to sunburn. Even embarrassment can cause some people to develop a rash.

Recommended supplements are a strong preparation of B complex vitamins, zinc and essential fatty acids.

See also **Acne** and **Eczema**.

R

SCHIZOPHRENIA

Schizophrenia is the name given to a number of vaguely understood diseases which affect the mind. It is said to affect one person in a hundred, mostly young people in their teens and in their twenties. In schizophrenia the mind is seriously disordered, and the patient's thoughts and behaviour lose touch with reality. Thinking becomes disjointed and emotions and reactions inappropriate to circumstances and surroundings. The schizophrenic has no perception of his own condition and finds his own behaviour perfectly acceptable. Other people's behaviour, by comparison, is not! Any one or more of the following symptoms may be present: disturbing conversation, distorted perceptions, persecution mania, hallucinations and delusions, bizarre thoughts, antisocial behaviour, 'hearing' voices, apparent inability to co-operate. The best thing is not to upset the patient – go along with him as much as you are able.

If these symptoms are acute the patient is said to be psychotic and therefore may require compulsory hospital treatment. It is unlikely that he will go willingly to see a doctor, and it is not always easy to find a doctor instantly available to visit the patient. In any case, if the doctor thinks that hospitalisation is required, he will need to call a psychiatrist to make out the necessary compulsory order for hospital treatment.

If you should ever find yourself in the unenviable position of dealing with a psychotic patient, and are having difficulty in obtaining the required medical attention in a hurry, I strongly recommend that you call the police and an ambulance. The chances are you will find them experienced and helpful and, even more to the point, they will arrive quickly. Until you can get help it is important to placate the patient.

Schizophrenia is due to a chemical imbalance and not, as some people have been told in the past, to inadequacies of upbringing. The tendency to develop schizophrenia is inherited. It is more common in those who suffer from coeliac disease. As coeliac disease is an adverse reaction to gluten, and schizophrenia is strongly linked to food sensitivity, this is not too surprising.

Trials have been done giving schizophrenics gluten-free/milk-free diets. On these diets many patients have improved dramatically and regressed when these same foods were re-introduced.

Schizophrenia has been strongly linked with food sensitivity by a number of doctors and therefore *any* food, or combination of foods, may be responsible. (People who are sensitive to one food only are in the minority.)

Dr. W. A. Hemmings, an immunologist at the University College of North Wales, commented in the *Lancet* as far back as 1978 that food allergy, especially to wheat, was a very likely cause of mental symptoms. Certainly, abnormally high amounts of antibodies to wheat and other foods have been found in the blood of schizophrenic patients. It is also

S

known now that we can become sensitive to our own *Candida* (a yeast in the gut flora), causing candidiasis which can cause mental symptoms in addition to physical ones.

Another possible cause is enzyme deficiencies. First of all we need to produce glucose. To obtain energy from glucose and oxygen we need enzymes to oxidise the glucose to carbon dioxide and water. Petrochemicals and other toxic matter in our environment poison the enzymes and cause abnormalities in the brain cells, leading to all manner of mental illnesses. Chemical transmitter systems in the brain are easily upset by toxic products and allergies. Schizophrenia can be the result of allergic reactions to foods and/or pollutants, enzyme deficiencies, toxic poisoning from heavy metals, or deficiencies of one or more trace minerals (very often zinc) or a combination of any of these factors.

So, after all that, you say, how can I ever begin to help a schizophrenic relative? In the short term you must be guided by the orthodox medical profession. A wide variety of drugs exist to calm the patient down, which is in his own interests as well as yours. Your biggest hurdle is to persuade him that he needs treatment. You may have to collaborate with his doctor and get him there on the pretence of a physical ailment. Your doctor, or, if in hospital, the consultant in charge, will choose whichever drug seems most appropriate in the circumstances. It is essential that the anti-psychotic medication normally used for schizophrenics is not withdrawn suddenly or the symptoms are very likely to return. Electro-convulsive therapy (ECT) is used for some forms of schizophrenia and has an immediate and calming effect on the patient.

New studies have been done to indicate the importance of zinc in brain function in the treatment of schizophrenia. Zinc is very often low in the mentally ill, as is folic acid. Such patients may also be deficient in one or more of the B vitamins. Earl Mindell, in *The Vitamin Bible*, tells of Dr Linus Pauling, Nobel Laureate of Stanford University, California, administering massive doses of vitamin C to schizophrenics in a series of tests to determine individual vitamin requirements and proving that they actually needed such high doses. Multiple digestive enzymes are also recommended as being helpful. The amino acid glutamine has been used successfully in the treatment of schizophrenia, and methionine, another amino acid, helps in some cases by lowering the level of histamine in the blood.

Foods which are likely causes of schizophrenia are wheat, other grains, milk and milk products, tea, coffee, citrus fruits, chocolate, alcohol, sugar, yeast, cola and other fizzy drinks, artificial additives, especially the azo and coal-tar dyes and the benzoates. Inhalant allergens implicated are airborne chemicals such as diesel fumes, tobacco smoke, perfumes and synthetic chemicals.

To anyone who has the misfortune to suffer from schizophrenia I would say this. Make a note of the above information and try to find a doctor specialising in nutrition to advise you on supplements. Cut out

S

the above foods (preferably with someone to help you), one at a time if you prefer, for a week or two remembering to re-introduce a very small amount initially and inform your family, friends and work colleagues of what you are doing and try to enlist their support. Try to check on any inhalants that cause your symptoms.

When you do find which foods adversely affect you, try hard not to succumb to the temptation of having them because once off your diet it is difficult for you to realize (or anyone else to get through to you) the importance of avoiding the foods or chemicals which affect you. It is not always easy avoiding inhalant allergens, I know. In fact you can be desensitised to both foods and inhalants through intradermal testing and neutralisation or EPD treatment (see Chapter 7) and there are, without doubt, some potentially schizophrenic patients around who keep their condition well under control by either of these methods. These symptoms are most distressing, and I wholeheartedly sympathise, but I do implore you to take responsibility for trying to stay well by whatever means you can – and this may require much willpower if allergies to foods are concerned – thereby saving yourself and your relatives untold distress.

SHAKING (TREMOR)

If you find that you cannot stop your hands, head or any other part of you from shaking, this means there is some imbalance between the action of the muscles and the nerves. It is not unnatural to start shaking if you become nervous or fearful or upset and angry, but you know from experience that this will disappear once you calm down. Shaking can also be a symptom of taking too much alcohol and also coming off it too abruptly. Again, you will return to normal after the toxic effects have worn off. As people get older they may become a little shaky but this is not what I am referring to here. I am concerned with a pronounced tremor which may have come on suddenly and could be allergy-induced. Certain non-allergic medical conditions, such as an over-active thyroid gland, for example, can cause shaking so it is essential to check with your doctor before assuming that it is of allergic origin.

I can find no documentation on the subject except in relation to caffeine sensitivity, but I know I developed this symptom on two separate occasions, first when coffee started affecting me and, at a later date, when I developed a cow's milk allergy. I have also heard of it being caused by a reaction to sugar. Therefore, should you develop a tremor, I suggest that you consider as possible causes all the caffeine-containing products – coffee, tea, chocolate and cola, followed by milk, sugar or any other commonly consumed foods. Watch out also for food additives; Patent Blue (E131) has been known to cause this symptom.

See also **Twitching**.

S

SHOULDER, STIFFNESS IN

Stiffness in a shoulder, if not caused by an injury, is usually due to fibrositis, especially if accompanied by pain in the neck. This type of rheumatic pain may be due to strain following over-use of the muscles. A short rest, plenty of heat and pain-killers will help to relieve the situation. Chronic conditions include a frozen shoulder (for which the cause is not known but which will eventually clear up of its own accord) as well as osteoarthritis and rheumatoid arthritis, both of which are often found to be allergic in origin.

Most likely causes are wheat, corn, milk, cheese, coffee, tea, yeast, chocolate, citrus fruits, sugar, pork, food additives, especially colourings, monosodium glutamate (MSG) and sodium nitrite.

See also **Arthritis** and **Neck Pain**.

SINUSITIS

Sinusitis is inflammation of the mucous membranes of the sinuses. The sinuses are air cavities in the skull bones lined with membranes linking up with those inside the nose. The symptoms include a headache over the eyes, an ache in the cheeks, catarrh, blocked nose and a lessened sense of taste and smell. If fever or severe pain should develop, call the doctor.

Sinusitis can develop from the catarrh which follows a cold or 'flu or it can be the result of persistent rhinitis. A headache when you get up in the morning, or which is most noticeable on bending down, is a likely sign of sinusitis.

Catarrh which follows a cold may last for a week or two but usually decreases gradually until it disappears altogether. It is advisable not to blow your nose too fiercely when you have a cold as this can force infection into the sinuses. Should this happen and your sinusitis get worse, your doctor can prescribe antibiotics if necessary.

Sinus headaches can also result from allergic rhinitis as the catarrh becomes trapped in the swollen nasal passages. Prolonged irritation of the nasal membranes can occasionally lead to nasal polyps.

Inhalations of steam from boiling water, with some added *Vick* or *Friar's Balsam*, will help to clear the nasal passages whatever the cause.

So, if you suffer from chronic sinusitis caused by allergic rhinitis what can you do? The answer is: look for the cause of the rhinitis. If it occurs only in the spring it may be caused by tree pollen; in the summer grass pollen, and late summer/early autumn, moulds. One can be desensitised against these allergens but they are seasonal, anyway, so they will cause only a temporary problem. That leaves us with foods and environmental allergens. The most likely foods are milk, wheat, cheese, citrus fruits, eggs, chocolate and food additives. Most likely inhalant allergens are tobacco smoke, perfumes, chemical pollution, dust, poorly ventilated, overheated

S

or damp atmospheres, or *excessive use of decongestant nose drops.*

One gramme of vitamin C taken three times a day is the most important supplement to help clear the sinuses.

See also **Catarrh** and **Nasal Polyps.**

SMELL, INCREASED SENSE OF

'If you can smell it, suspect it' was some very good advice given by a clinical ecologist doctor who was speaking to a chemically-sensitive audience.

A number of people have problems in this direction and it makes life very difficult for them. Their sense of smell is usually very acute, and it may require only the most minute amount of an inhalant to make them ill. Such people pick up smells long before the average person. A friend who lives nearby has an arrangement with our local pharmaceutical company whereby *she* will inform *them* when their waste product fumes become unacceptably high! There are also some people for whom the odours of cooking foods – fish and eggs being typical examples – are enough to set off allergic reactions.

An expert on formaldehyde, speaking at a conference, said that sensitive people could react to as little as one part in four million of formaldehyde; this seems quite incredible, but it gives us some idea of what these unfortunate individuals may be up against. Short of living in a bubble it is almost impossible in this day and age not to come into contact with chemical pollutants.

Pregnant women, especially those who are allergic, can develop an increased sense of smell, albeit temporary. I suspect that their altered hormone balance causes them to become more susceptible to inhalant allergens.

Some household smells which are better avoided, or at least satisfactorily substituted, are smoke, fumes from gas and oil-fired central heating, detergents, washing powders, household cleaners and air fresheners.

See also **Pregnancy, Advice on.**

SMELL AND TASTE, LACK OF SENSE OF

Hay fever and sinusitis sufferers are likely to have a diminished sense of smell, especially if they develop nasal polyps. Allergic children who are permanently snuffly may have a poor sense of smell and taste, which may account for why many of them are faddy eaters.

Sometimes people develop a loss of sense of smell and taste (the two usually go together) following a brain operation. On other occasions there is no apparent reason, but the situation causes much distress. Such people have sometimes been found to be very deficient in zinc – not surprising considering that most zinc which occurs naturally in foods is lost in processing. In order for zinc to work most efficiently it should be accompanied by vitamin A, calcium and phosphorus supplements.

S

SORE THROAT

A sore throat, uncomfortable but common, frequently accompanies a cold, 'flu or other infections. It is the main symptom of tonsilitis where the tonsils become infected or inflamed. Sometimes the larynx may become inflamed and this causes the voice to become husky, possibly little more than a whisper. Either of these complaints may require an antibiotic.

An allergy to foods or inhalants can also cause sore throats which may lead to tonsilitis or laryngitis. Other symptoms which may accompany an allergy-induced sore throat or, indeed, be present on their own, are mucus in the throat, difficulty in swallowing, catarrh, cough, dry throat or a feeling of a 'lump in the throat'.

Sometimes people suffer from constant sore throats and, until allergy is considered, may never find the cause. My husband suffered this way for months, if not years, and the whole family were checked (with negative results) to see whether they were carriers. Even his secretary was examined, but to no avail! The doctor professed himself mystified. As soon as we moved, his sore throats disappeared. I strongly suspect that they were related to the pesticide sprayed regularly on the produce in the market garden over the road from where we lived.

Possible allergens include foods, among the most common being milk, wheat and eggs, but very many sore throats are caused by inhalant allergens – the most likely being car exhaust fumes, gas fumes, cigarette smoke, paint, cleaning fluids, perfumes, disinfectants, air fresheners, aerosol sprays, pesticides and air pollution generally.

I recommend the following supplements for people susceptible to sore throats and allied symptoms, whatever the cause: vitamin C (1g daily, or 3g daily whilst sore throat is severe), vitamin A, vitamin E and garlic perles. The latter are small capsules which are easily swallowed and give off no odour.

STINGS, BEE AND WASP

Bee or wasp stings are usually painful at first and then become itchy. In addition to swelling, inflammation and itching, they can cause fever, nausea, fainting and nettlerash (and sometimes blisters may occur) if the individual is allergic to the venom. The symptoms may be anything from very mild to very severe. If scratching can be avoided so much the better, because if the area becomes infected the symptoms will intensify and spread.

In a severe allergic reaction to a bee or wasp sting the swelling will come on quickly. In rare cases there is an acute allergic reaction to the sting's poison, causing a massive release of histamine where the patient may find it hard to breathe or, indeed, may collapse. A very small number of people die each year, usually from bee stings, *but this is very rare*.

S

Seek immediate medical help if the patient is stung in the mouth or throat, if breathing becomes difficult, if his joints, tongue or lips begin to swell, if itching and/or swelling begins to spread, or if there are any other symptoms of allergic reaction.

When there is no allergic reaction, home treatment is as follows. Clean the area with antiseptic and bathe with water to relieve itching. Treat with calamine lotion or *Anthisan*. (Not for more than a day or two for the latter as you can develop an allergy to it.) For a wasp sting, treat with vinegar or other astringent, and for a bee sting treat with sodium bicarbonate mixed to a paste with water. If the patient is subject to allergies, give an antihistamine.

Wasps hardly ever sting if left alone but may do so when people get over-excited. Bees are more likely to sting, especially when they get dozy. Both are attracted to foods – particularly sugar, jams and honey – and picnics are the most notorious places for stings to occur. Insect repellent creams can be bought, but sensitive people can be allergic to them.

If you have ever had a severe reaction to a bee or wasp sting, ask your doctor whether he would recommend you being desensitised to bee and wasp venom. This is worth considering and it is a service available under the NHS. Alternatively, he may wish to prescribe for you a 'Medihaler Epi' inhaler which contains adrenalin and which should therefore be used only for *emergency* treatment. He may prefer to prescribe for you an effective antihistamine tablet which you should always carry on your person to protect yourself in the event of being stung.

High doses of vitamin C and B complex vitamins are said to protect against a severe reaction to a bee or wasp sting; I found this interesting to learn when I researched the subject, as these vitamins are also highly effective for protection against other forms of allergic reaction.

See also **Anaphylactic Shock**.

STOOLS, BLOOD IN

This distressing symptom may be indicative of a serious condition and should be reported to your doctor at once. I can find no reference to blood in the stools in my 'library' of books on allergy. However, I have had a small number of proven cases reported where blood in the stools accompanied other symptoms in an allergic reaction. Therefore, if your doctor decides that you are in good general health, and neither he nor you consider the situation warrants further investigation, or if investigation does not turn up any other cause, you may care to look to your diet, especially if you already know you are food-allergic.

See also **Ulcerative Colitis**.

STRESS

'Stress' must be one of the most over-used words in the English language today. I wonder just how many people complain to their doctors of fatigue/overwork/worry/depression. The doctor nods wisely and says 'You are suffering from stress', as he reaches for the prescription pad to prescribe yet another tranquilliser. One cannot generalise, of course; not all doctors are like this. In fairness to them, how can they possibly discuss the patient's problems and life-style in the five minutes allocated to them in the average surgery visit? Yet this is what is needed – someone to listen, someone to help put the problems in perspective, someone to offer wise, objective advice. This is why half the American population have their own personal analysts. We may laugh but it seems to me to be an excellent idea. In any case, whatever the Americans come up with is usually adopted by the British some years later.

Everyone suffers from stress at some time in their lives, and some people for much of their lives. Often it is through no fault of their own. Others cause their own stress by adopting a life-style which can lead only to disaster. Many stresses we impose upon ourselves. Apart from wars which cause anguish and suffering to the masses, and murder, rape and other crimes which do the same to individuals, much of our everyday stress is due to our inability to relate to one another.

However, there is another form of stress, and that is the stress of food and chemical allergy. If this were recognised as an important aspect of health, and patients were told of its relevance to chronic ill-health and how it can affect their outlook on life, not only would it encourage them to take more responsibility for their own health but it would leave doctors free to concentrate on patients with other serious medical problems. A growing number of doctors do recognise this, and their patients have good reason to be grateful to them.

One of the major stresses in the western world since World War II has been the increasing use of chemicals in our environment and the pollution this has brought in its wake. So many chemicals have been introduced into our food and atmosphere that no one knows precisely just how many; however, the number runs into many thousands, and it is ever on the increase. Each new unnatural substance we come across poses a stress as the body tries to adapt to it. In some areas there are pockets of pollution which stress people's bodies to breaking point, so that ill-health results. Some food factories resemble chemistry laboratories as they churn out additive-filled, artificially-flavoured, chemically-preserved processed foods. Each successive generation finds it yet harder to adapt.

The good news is that things *are* beginning to change. Those people who, for years, have been concerned about such matters are banding together to give voice and *at last* they are being heard. The subject of environmental illness *will* be introduced into medical training. The Government is being *forced* into taking action and is making some attempt to reverse the damage we have done to our environment and therefore ourselves, so there is reason to be optimistic.

See also **Anxiety, Depression, Nervousness** and **Panic Attacks**.

S

TENSION/FATIGUE SYNDROME

The tension/fatigue syndrome, a classic allergy condition, is so called because the patient is both tense and exhausted. Although the sufferer desperately needs rest and peace and quiet, his over-working brain will not allow this. Tension/fatigue syndrome is common in both children and adults.

Children with this problem usually look 'run-down' and have dark circles under their eyes, known as 'allergic shiners'. They may suffer any combination of the following symptoms: drowsiness, inability to concentrate, confusion, depression, anxiety, inability to keep still, inability to sleep, hyperactivity, poor co-ordination, over-emotion and temper tantrums. Some children will be more prone to drowsiness, others to hyperactivity. Either way, life is not easy for them, especially as they will be constantly in trouble for symptoms which are beyond their control. This will sap their self-confidence and affect their whole psychological development.

Adults who have this problem suffer from similar symptoms – fatigue, confusion, inability to concentrate, nervousness, mental exhaustion, over excitement and possibly even violent mood swings. They may be diagnosed as neurotic or worse, mentally disturbed, and may be sent to see a psychiatrist – which will do no good whatsoever if it is their diet or environment which is at fault. People who go on to elimination diets to try to track down their physical symptoms often find, to their delight, that any mental symptoms (for which they may have blamed themselves) disappear alongside the physical ones – only to reappear when the culprit foods (or inhalants) are re-introduced. In some people the symptoms are constant, in others they are spasmodic. So called 'Monday morning blues' are usually a hangover from something eaten or drunk over the weekend.

Child or adult, to be constantly exhausted and yet unable to sleep because your brain is rushing around in circles in an apparently endless succession is like being on a merry-go-round which never ceases. 'Stop the world – I want to get off' perhaps best describes the desperation of the unfortunate sufferer.

The foods most commonly responsible are those which contain caffeine, ie coffee, tea, chocolate, cola and over-the-counter caffeine-containing medications. Individual reactions are most likely to be to milk, wheat, eggs, cheese, citrus fruits, spices and artificial additives.

I strongly recommend a multi-vitamin/multi-mineral supplement, high in B vitamins, and 1g of vitamin C daily to help to boost up the immune system.

Finally, please do not forget that any of the symptoms mentioned, either for children or adults, can be related to other illnesses so, if in doubt, do consult your doctor. Although one frequently hears of the medical profession missing allergies as a cause of illness, it is not

T

unknown for symptoms to be assumed to be of allergic origin when, in fact, they are not.

See also **Myalgic Encephalomyelitis (ME)**, **Fatigue**.

THYROID DISORDERS

People who suffer from food allergies to any degree usually have a problem with hypoglycaemia, and as blood sugar levels are related to the thyroid hormone, it is easy to deduce that there may be a connection between food allergies and the thyroid gland.

Some people already know that certain foods or chemical inhalants cause their thyroid gland to become over-stimulated, causing an increase in the gland's secretion. If this condition persists, thyroid function tests can be done. If these prove positive, anti-thyroid drugs may be prescribed. Alternatively, some of the thyroid gland may be removed and, if necessary, replacement thyroid given to provide the right balance. A doctor's advice is essential, and a second opinion from an endocrinologist is advisable; with treatment, the prognosis is excellent.

However, if you develop a thyroid condition and you are a known allergy sufferer, do remind your doctor of this because there are two further possibilities. You may be having an allergic reaction to something which is over-stimulating your thyroid gland – in which case discovering and removing the offending item will be sufficient to regulate your thyroid gland. Alternatively, it is possible to have allergic reactions which cause symptoms that *simulate* hypothyroidism or hyperthyroidism when, in fact, the relevant tests prove negative. Either way, suspect first the caffeine-containing products coffee, tea, chocolate and cola, especially if taken in excess. Erythrosine (E127) is known to cause hyperthyroidism when taken in large amounts. Certain chemical inhalants are capable of producing the same effect.

TINNITUS (NOISES IN THE EAR)

Noises in the ear may be described as ringing, buzzing, humming, roaring or tinkling – different noises, presumably, to different people! What they do have in common is that they are not caused by an external factor but by an internal, physical one. There are a variety of possible causes. It may be due to the hardening of one of the small bones in the ear or growth on the nerve of the ear, in fact, any damage to the hearing mechanism may result in tinnitus.

More common reasons, however, are catarrh or ear wax. Ear wax can be removed at the surgery by syringing but the patient is advised to soften the wax with warm olive oil or something similar for a few days beforehand. When tinnitus is accompanied by giddiness and deafness it is known as Ménière's disease. This is also allergic in origin. People who suffer from high blood pressure may be conscious of a pulsating sound in

T

the ear; the sound will disappear with the correct treatment. A number of drugs, including aspirin in large doses, can cause a ringing in the ears.

Tinnitus is a common symptom of people constantly exposed to loud noise. This applies particularly to people in the world of pop music who, for the last few decades, have felt it necessary to extend the volume way above the recommended decibels. Not surprisingly, many are experiencing irreversible deafness at a relatively early age. Exposure to *one* instance of an *intensely* loud noise can cause sufficient damage to cause tinnitus.

Tinnitus which appears 'for no apparent reason' is almost invariably due to the effects of food or inhaled chemical allergies. I believe that many people may experience this to a minor degree without ever being aware of it. Incredible though it may seem, I was well into middle age before I realised that 'silence' did not mean a mild and unobtrusive humming noise! Now I have worked out my allergies, I rather miss it!

This symptom is frequently referred to in allergy books but I can find no documentation regarding possible allergens so I suggest investigating first those which are most common among foods, food additives and chemical inhalants.

See also **Ménière's Disease**.

'TODDLER DIARRHOEA'

Acute diarrhoea can be caused by contaminated water or food poisoning due to bacterial or viral infection, so a doctor should be consulted immediately where a small child is involved.

Persistent diarrhoea of a less acute nature should also be checked out in case infection is present.

'Toddler diarrhoea' is a phrase which has crept into medical jargon in recent years. It is used when a doctor cannot explain its presence. Many mothers are told: 'This is quite normal, do not worry, he will grow out of it.' I say it is *not* normal. You should worry, and he will outgrow it only if the rate at which he develops outweighs the severity of his allergic response – otherwise he may get worse. The answer lies with his diet. The one exception is that 'toddler diarrhoea' can be due to a lack of enzymes rather than to an allergic reaction. This may be due to the child's immaturity – in which case he will grow out of it – or it may be a congenital deficiency which will be with him for life. Whichever cause, the dietary approach will save much unnecessary stress for both mother and infant, and offending foods can be tested again at a later stage.

Either way, then, there is something in the child's diet to which he is sensitive and, with a youngster, this is not too difficult to detect. Try to think back to when the problem started and see if you can relate it to the introduction of a new food or drink. The most common cause is cow's milk and if the child has had this symptom since birth, or shortly after (if he was bottle fed), or shortly after you weaned him onto cow's milk (if he was breast-fed) then there is your answer. There are also

T

some babies whose sensitivity to cow's milk is severe enough for them to be affected by traces of the allergen in their mother's breast-milk. If this proves to be the case, then it would be wise for *you* to give up cow's milk (and its products) for the time being and continue breast-feeding. The only alternative is to change to one of the brands of soya milk made especially for babies.

If you get no joy with this line of thought think also what else he had as an infant – orange juice, sugar, honey? Regarding a young baby, say under six months of age, he may simply be unable to tolerate a new food because his digestive and immune systems are just too immature to cope with it. In this case it is far better that he is well on his formula alone and that other foods are delayed until he can cope with them (although pureed fruits and vegetables should be safe in most cases). I am glad to say that the fashion of putting babies onto solids as early as possible is fading fast because it has been responsible for many infants developing sensitivities who otherwise would not have done so.

For a weaned child with 'toddler diarrhoea' I suggest removing all processed foods and putting him onto a natural diet of pure foods and, if this does not do the trick, each food will have to be tested on an individual basis. I would strongly recommend that processed foods containing artificial additives not be given to children of any age – but particularly not to young ones. The child may even be affected by your water supply if you live in an area where this is not too pure. If you suspect this, it can easily be proved one way or another by replacing temporarily with bottled water. If you *do* find that your water is responsible, then a water filter can be bought from health food or hardware shops at no great cost.

If no medical explanation can be given for 'toddler diarrhoea' then the answer is among those things he eats and drinks, and everything that goes into his mouth (including toothpaste and vitamin drops) must be taken into consideration. You *will* find the answer if you persevere, for, most surely, there is one.

See also **Diarrhoea**.

TONGUE, CONDITIONS OF THE

T

The tongue is rather like a barometer in that it gives a certain indication of the state of our health. The tongue of a healthy, non-smoker should be clean, pink and moist, and it should be covered in small, raised areas. A smooth tongue can be a sign of anaemia. The tongue tends to become furred in a feverish condition. Ulcers on the tongue may be due to infection or allergy.

In allergic reactions many people experience tingling or numbness of the tongue. In a severe allergic reaction the tongue and lips can swell very rapidly to many times their normal size. This can happen in the case of a bee sting, for example.

Other allergens which can produce this same result are certain foods, those most commonly documented being eggs, peanuts and gluten (found in wheat, oats, barley and rye). Even the most minute amounts can cause a severe reaction of this nature, and rapid medical help is essential. If in doubt, call both an ambulance and your doctor.

See also **Mouth Ulcers** and **Stings**.

TRAVEL SICKNESS (MOTION SICKNESS)

Motion sickness can be caused by travel by road, sea or air. Few people suffer from sickness in an aircraft or on a ship on a smooth journey. Fewer still have problems when travelling by train. By and large car sickness is the major problem, so I shall concentrate on this.

The orthodox explanation is that when the balancing mechanism of the ear is altered by the motion of the vehicle, the brain is affected in a way which causes nausea. The constant motion gives no relief until such time as the journey is over.

The ecologist's or environmentalist's view is that the nausea is much more likely to be due to an individual sensitivity either to the inhalation of other people's exhaust fumes or the phenol 'outgassing' of the plastic fabrics used in the car upholstery and the inside body work which continue to give off fumes long after their manufacture. In cars upholstered in leather, there is the problem of the tanning chemicals with which the leather has been treated. Either of these can produce a wide range of symptoms in susceptible people, nausea being a common one. There may be other causes, too, or a reaction may be due to a combination of causes.

There is much which can be done to give the sensitive person his best chance of symptom-free travel. If you or one of your passengers is in this category, I make the following suggestions:

1. Take only a light meal with no alcohol before travelling.
2. Take a sickness pill half to one hour before your journey is due to start.
3. Put on sufficient clothing in order to have some fresh air circulating at all times and still be warm.
4. Advise sufferer to sit next to a window and keep looking out.
5. Plan in advance for time for stops.
6. Don't allow sufferer to read or do anything which requires looking down.
7. Do not allow smoking in the car.
8. Take barley sugars, glucose tablets or something similar.
9. When behind other vehicles in slow traffic, close windows. The larger the vehicle the greater the fumes! Keep your distance.
10. Try, if you can, to avoid travelling in the vicinity of roads being tarred, pesticide spraying, factory pollution and so on. (An open sunroof probably allows in a smaller amount of fumes than does an open window.)

T

11. If you are the driver, do not take *any* antihistamine which is known to cause drowsiness. *Triludan* or *Hismanal* should be alright.
12. If you are the driver, and you begin to feel sleepy, *do* stop the car at the first available parking spot, get out, and take a short walk – taking deep breaths of fresh air.

TWITCHING (NERVOUS TIC)

This is spasmodic and involuntary contraction and relaxation of the muscles and can apply to any part of the body. Sometimes it is the eyelids or a muscle in the face, shoulder or a limb. It is a common complaint, and children and the elderly are particularly susceptible. It may be hereditary or may accompany a disorder of the nervous system, but the general orthodox view is that it is a stress symptom and can be caused by insecurity or anxiety. This explanation does not account for the number of people in whom this symptom occurs for no apparent reason. If it is due to a nervous reaction then the twitching is best ignored, as drawing attention to it is only likely to make it worse. However, it is important to discover whether anything *is* worrying the child. Either way, the twitching will probably disappear after a few months – so say the orthodox medical books. However, what if it does *not* disappear?

Involuntary restlessness of the limbs is a similar affliction. The legs, especially, may become restless, perhaps more so in the evening or after going to bed – which can make for a disturbed night.

Both of these conditions are not uncommon allergic reactions of the nervous system, and the most likely causes are caffeine-containing foods – coffee, tea, chocolate and cola. Artificial colourings and other additives are also suspect. Any other foods could be equally responsible. Restless legs are often the result of consuming caffeine. The problem may be aggravated by a lack of magnesium, so I recommend taking this as a supplement.

T

ULCERATIVE COLITIS

Ulcerative colitis is inflammation of the colon (large bowel) which leads to ulceration. It is usually accompanied by abdominal pain, bloody diarrhoea and mucus. Attacks may be mild, with pain low in the abdomen, or sudden and severe with blood and mucus in the stools. At its worst, severe diarrhoea consisting of water, blood and pus may occur up to twenty times daily. There may be alternating diarrhoea and constipation with abdominal pain. This can be localised or spread, and can involve the whole colon. Haemorrhage is not uncommon. Fever, loss of appetite, loss of weight and anaemia are all additional possibilities.

If ulcers perforate the bowel, severe abdominal pain will occur, requiring immediate medical attention. If ulcerative colitis starts in childhood and progresses well into adulthood, there is a high risk of developing cancer of the bowel, but the risk is greatly reduced with proper treatment.

The orthodox recommendation is to 'eat a normal diet, other than cutting out raw fruits and vegetable roughage', to rest, to take anti-diarrhoea preparations and to avoid stress (rather ironic when the ulcerative colitis is by far the most stressful aspect to your life!).

A doctor should always be consulted in this highly distressing and incapacitating illness, especially if the symptoms are rapidly worsening or recurrent bouts are extended. In these circumstances your doctor may send you for a barium enema and internal examination, or may prescribe drugs to lessen attacks – these may well be some form of steroid – and/or he may 'advise a suitable diet' or, in severe cases, he may advise an ileostomy. In this operation the colon is removed and the ileum (small bowel) extended to an opening in the abdomen where it empties into special disposable bags attached to the skin.

On average, ten per cent of sufferers recover, ten per cent get worse with serious complications, and the others carry on in much the same way with good and bad times. The orthodox view is that the cause is unknown. This is in spite of all the trials done over the years showing that ulcerative colitis may be (and very often is) of allergic origin. Some patients already have recognised allergic symptoms such as eczema, hay fever or asthma. They quite often suffer from mouth ulcers as well.

Ulcerative colitis has long been believed to be due to neurosis because of the accompanying symptoms of fatigue, weakness, nervousness and irritability (all classic allergy symptoms); unfortunate patients of the past – and doubtless some of the present day – have been prescribed bland, milky diets when milk has frequently, in scientifically controlled trials, been proved to be the incriminating factor. (You would think that when doctors saw their patients deteriorating on these diets this might tell them something!)

In the 1920s Dr Albert Rowe, an allergist in San Francisco, put patients with colitis on exclusion diets with considerable success. In

U

1942 Dr A. F. R. Andresen, in the American Journal of Digestive Disease, considered that ulcerative colitis was often due to food allergy, with milk being the incriminating factor. In the 1950s Dr Ted Randolph of Chicago gave his colitis patients nothing but spring water until their symptoms subsided and also found considerable success. Dr Richard Mackarness, in his book *Not all in the Mind*, refers to Professor Truelove of Oxford 'confirming verbally to me his findings on the role of milk provoking attacks of ulcerative colitis' and thanks him for 'permission to quote from his published work on the subject in the BMJ'.

It must not be thought that milk is the only food capable of causing these horrific symptoms. It is simply the most common one. Many doctors have failed by putting patients onto a milk-free diet alone because, even when milk *is* involved there are often several other foods responsible too in the same patient. In other patients possibly only one food may be involved but this is not necessarily milk.

More recently, Dr Len McEwen, who developed the enzyme-potentiated desensitisation vaccine (EPD for short) for allergy sufferers has found this to be helpful in those patients suffering from colitis and has written details of his trial in the medical journal *Clinical Ecology*.

Those doctors who perform a colostomy or ileostomy on their patients before considering the strong possibility of the symptoms being of allergic origin are subjecting them to irreversible and mutilating operations which can have devastating psychological consequences.

Even infants can suffer from colitis, though this is comparatively rare, and here the cause is cow's milk in the great majority of cases; their main symptom is diarrhoea containing blood and mucus. If the baby is bottle-fed then changing to a soya-based formula should solve the problem. If the baby is breast-fed then the mother will need to eliminate whatever food/foods are causing her baby's symptoms. Cow's milk is the most likely so she will need to cut cow's milk out and all its products as well. If her baby does not improve, then wheat and eggs are the next most suspect, and so on. If the mother has difficulty in isolating the culprit foods but still wants to breast-feed, she can discuss with her doctor the possibility of Nalcrom (sodium cromoglycate) being prescribed to her. This is the food-allergy-blocking agent. It has a good safety record and is not absorbed into the blood stream but gets eliminated in the natural way in due course.

Now, back to ulcerative colitis in general. What are the foods most likely to be responsible? They are cow's milk (by far the most common), wheat, eggs, coffee, tea, chocolate, cola, citrus fruits, cheese, chicken, potatoes and tomatoes. You can consider chemical pollution too because *all* allergy-induced conditions can be caused or worsened by this; however, this is not so regularly documented.

How can you be helped? First of all you *must* go onto an elimination diet (see Chapter 5) to discover which foods are responsible. If you can do this under the supervision of a doctor working in this field so much

U

the better, but it is not essential. When you have sorted out your diet (which will be individual and suited to the requirements of your own body), you can consider the following advice.

Try to avoid emotional stress. This is *not* a cause of ulcerative colitis but will certainly aggravate it. Lack of vitamin K causes colitis, and you will find this in yoghurt, egg yolk, safflower, soya bean and fish liver oils, green leafy vegetables and the supplements alfalfa and kelp. However, do note that Earl Mindell, in *The Vitamin Bible*, says: '...if you are taking an anti-coagulant be aware that this vitamin (even in natural foods) can reverse the drug's effects.' You will also benefit from additional vitamin U which is to be found in raw cabbage, cabbage juice and alfalfa also.

Take plenty of water – six to eight glasses daily. The purity of water varies from area to area. Even where the water is very pure, some people are affected by the chlorine. If you find you are better on bottled water you may decide to invest in a water filter. Also recommended are acidophilus (3–6 capsules daily) and a teaspoonful of bran flakes daily (if you are not wheat-allergic), but the most valuable aids of all are the alfalfa and kelp tablets which you will find in health food shops.

UNCONSCIOUSNESS

There are many causes of a loss of consciousness. Unconsciousness occurs as a result of a poor blood supply to the brain. Some such causes are heart conditions, pregnancy, loss of blood, excessive standing (particularly in hot weather) or simply the fragility of old age. The patient will become very pale and start sweating before collapsing. His pulse will be found to be weak and his blood pressure low.

Very allergic people may go into a state of shock, known as anaphylactic shock, and collapse after a bee or other insect sting or after consuming even a minute amount of food to which they are highly sensitive. Those foods most likely to cause this are fish, shellfish, eggs, nuts and peanuts. The same thing can happen as the result of an acute allergic reaction to a medicine, notably penicillin. Also, some anaesthetics can cause anaphylactic shock, and even death, in susceptible people. Severely allergic people, therefore, should undertake an operation only after very careful consultation with the family doctor, prospective surgeon and anaesthetist. In a severe reaction, high levels of IgE (the antibody produced by allergy) are found in blood tissues. The mast cells explode, releasing large amounts of histamine, the body chemical which causes allergic symptoms.

The standard treatment for unconsciousness and collapse due to allergy is a shot of adrenalin or the administration of oxygen.

See also **Anaphylactic Shock, Fainting,** and **Stings**.

U

URTICARIA (NETTLERASH/HIVES)

Urticaria is recognised by a characteristic blistering or wealing of the skin surface. Histamine is released, causing blood vessels to dilate and leak fluid into the tissues causing swelling and red, itchy blotches. The weals and surrounding skin are intensely itchy. It looks like a sting from a nettle (hence the name 'nettlerash') and can affect any part of the body; it varies in size from a pin-prick to a large patch several inches (five or more centimetres) in diameter. It is a common condition, especially in children, and is normally accompanied by other symptoms which are allergic in origin – such as vomiting, abdominal pain and wheezing with diarrhoea to follow. Urticaria may cause swelling of face, limbs and joints. When it affects facial features, they can look quite alarming owing to the excessive swelling of the skin. The mouth, tongue and throat may swell and obstruct breathing. When the symptoms are particularly severe the condition known as giant hives or angioedema.

Some doctors believe that infectious, parasitic infestations and toxic conditions can cause urticaria. However, it is recognised – even by the most orthodox of doctors – as being due to an allergy or sensitivity in the great majority of cases. These fall into four categories: contact allergies, food allergies, inhalant allergies and physical sensitivities.

Contact allergies are caused by an allergic reaction when an allergen comes into contact with the patient's skin. These are known as contactants, and among the most likely are jewellery (usually nickel), clothing, animal danders and chemicals. Touching certain foods – such as shellfish, strawberries, egg whites (or egg shells) and nuts – may also give rise to the condition.

The food allergens (ie those allergens which are *eaten*) most often associated with urticaria are milk, eggs, shellfish, fish, nuts, chocolate, cheese, yeast, strawberries, wheat, tomatoes, peas and pork. Food additives can also be responsible, and frequently are. Watch out for E102, E110, E122, E123, E131, E132, E133, E142, 155, E160(b), E200, E210–E220, E223. This list includes the azo and coal-tar dyes, the benzoate preservatives and sulphur dioxide. Certain medicines, especially aspirin and penicillin, have been found to cause urticaria too. (People who are sensitive to penicillin may react to milk and beef also, as penicillin is frequently given to cows.)

Inhalant allergens are another possible cause of urticaria. Highly sensitive people can even react to the odours from foods as they are being cooked. Typical examples of these are fish and eggs, and it is even known for people to react adversely after *kissing* people who have recently consumed these foods. (Such is the life of the very allergic individual!) Other common inhalant allergens are air pollution, gas, aerosol sprays, smoke, car exhaust fumes, perfumes, paint, polish and formaldehyde – and doubtless many others.

U

A physical sensitivity is not an allergy as such but is likely to affect the same type of person. Urticaria can be caused, therefore, by pressure on the skin (weals may be drawn on the skin surface), exercise, sun, extremes of temperature, and even emotions such as fear and excitement.

Urticaria, whatever the cause, may appear in two distinct forms. It may come as an acute and dramatic reaction occurring very soon after contact with the allergen – which is most likely to be a food, penicillin or insect sting; in these cases, the cause is usually fairly obvious, and the symptoms will probably have disappeared within twenty-four hours. Alternatively, urticaria in its chronic form may continue for several days or even up to three weeks after the cause has been removed. One of the most soothing treatments is to dab calamine lotion onto the affected parts.

Consult your doctor if the itching is very intense, or if severe swelling appears, especially swelling of the mouth, tongue or throat or if there is a feeling of tightness in the chest. If there is difficulty in breathing, an injection of adrenalin can be given or corticosteroids prescribed. Antihistamines such as *Piriton* are sometimes used, but others such as *Hismanal* are less likely to produce side-effects and do not cause drowsiness.

Anyone subject to urticaria is obviously likely to be a rather allergic person and, as such, would benefit from taking supplements on a regular basis. Recommended are vitamin A, a strong preparation of B complex vitamins, vitamin C (1g daily), vitamin E, and a good multi-mineral. I would suggest that 1g of vitamin C is taken three times daily whilst the urticaria is at its most severe.

See also **Angioedema**.

VAGINAL DISCHARGE

Once a girl reaches puberty, and hormonal changes take place, it is normal for her to produce a creamy-white discharge from her vagina. This is likely to increase during pregnancy or on the Pill. Spotting of blood sometimes occurs also in the first two months after starting the Pill. These discharges are quite normal but other discharges require medical investigation.

An ectopic pregnancy (where the egg has not reached the womb but has attached itself to one of the Fallopian tubes) causes a brown discharge or slight bleeding and requires urgent medical attention. However, this is *very* rare and these symptoms can have a variety of less serious causes.

Discharge caused by venereal infection also needs fairly urgent attention. However, the possibility of having been infected by venereal disease is remote unless a girl or her partner have been promiscuous.

Other forms of infection may be unrelated to sexual intercourse. A common one is thrush – known medically as candidiasis. This produces a thick, white discharge and itching around the vulva and vagina. It can be caused by taking the Pill or too many antibiotics; it can also be present during pregnancy or can be caught from a sexual partner.

A discharge is quite commonly due to a condition known as vaginitis; this involves inflammation of the vagina which causes itching and soreness as well. Children and older women are prone to vaginitis because they have low oestrogen levels. The discharge may take any form, depending on the cause – which is likely to be a sensitivity to a deodorant, perfume, soap or talcum powder, or sometimes to sanitary towels or tampons. A very offensive discharge can be caused by a forgotten tampon. Vaginitis can also be due to thrush, in which case it will be known as thrush vaginitis.

Any abnormal discharge, whatever the cause, must be medically investigated – and the sooner the better. No one need feel embarrassed in discussing this in confidence with their doctor, who, in any case, will have heard it from patients many times before. A doctor once told me that about one woman in five will have this problem. I imagine the numbers will have risen dramatically due to the increase in thrush over recent years. Your doctor will probably wish to take a swab and do a urine test. For anyone who has not had a swab taken before, I can assure you that it is a simple and painless procedure.

If no infection can be found, then your vaginal discharge is most likely to be caused by a sensitivity. The same applies to cystitis and other genitourinary symptoms (including frequent urination and bed-wetting in children) when these are not associated with infection. This particularly applies when other symptoms of allergy are already present. People who suffer from gut and mucous membrane allergies are the most likely to be prone to allergy-related vaginal problems.

V

Sensitivity may be to things such as deodorants, perfumes, soaps and powders, as mentioned before. If plenty of baths and showers are taken it is quite unnecessary to use any of these direct. They are all, including soap, too harsh for such a delicate area. A sensitivity to sanitary towels and tampons is more of a problem but, by trying different brands, it should be possible to find one which suits you.

Last, but by no means least, it is very important to realise that vaginal discharge can be, and very often is, caused by an allergic reaction to certain foods. This is often referred to in books on food allergy but my research has not uncovered any reference as to likely culprits. Therefore, I suggest that you investigate first those which are known to be the most likely – milk, wheat, eggs etc.

Dr Jonathan Brostoff, in his book *The Complete Guide to Food Allergy and Intolerance*, tells of the migraine trial carried out on children at London's Great Ormond Street Hospital in 1982/3. The children chosen suffered from a wide variety of other symptoms as well as migraine. They were put on to a strict elimination diet. The doctors involved found that the most unexpected aspect of the trial was the way in which not only the migraine but the other symptoms – including vaginal discharge – cleared up by this method.

See also **Cystitis** and **Candidiasis**.

VIOLENCE

We live in violent times. We live in times where many ordinary citizens find it hard to understand the workings of the legal mind. Commonsense does not always seem to enter into our scheme of things.

Why does someone who has abused a woman, maybe a child, so often appear to get off with a light sentence and an admonition that he has been a naughty boy and it must not happen again? At the same time, it is totally unacceptable for a woman to use so much as a nail file in self defence of such an act? The same question applies regarding people who are brutally attacked or mugged. If they bring forth some weapon of self-defence, they may well find themselves in court being told that they must not take the law into their own hands. If the real criminals were to get heavy sentences for unprovoked attacks, there might be some sense in such an attitude, but so often they do not.

Television must take some responsibility for increased violence. On the one hand it is an excellent medium for bringing us so many interesting and entertaining programmes. On the other hand we have an obsession, seemingly, with producing films portraying killing, sadism and oppressive promiscuity. On screen, criminals are not infrequently made into heroes. Viewing such material, I believe, has a strong influence on the minds of certain people, especially some who have not lived through less violent times. For them this is the norm. If it is all they have ever viewed, possibly from an early age, and if they, in all innocence, take

V

these films at face value, is it surprising that they may be influenced by what they have seen?

These are personal views. Not everyone will agree with them. The following, however, is fact. Too much (or a sensitivity to) alcohol can lead to violence – as can drug-taking or inhaling solvents. We all know this – or at least most people are aware of it. What many people do not know is that some foods (such as sugar), chemicals in foods (such as azo dyes) and certain chemical inhalants can cause allergic reactions in susceptible people which will result in (or contribute to) aggression and even violent behaviour. In the majority of cases, when this happens, neither the allergy sufferer nor those around him will realise this, and no one will therefore be in a position to prevent it happening again.

However, allergies affecting the brain are recognised by doctors working in the field of environmental illness; these doctors are aware that the consequences of brain allergy can land a patient in court.

This therefore poses the question: can someone be held responsible for violent action perpetrated when suffering from a chemical imbalance? If the fair answer is 'no' then how many real criminals are going to plead: 'I was suffering from an allergic reaction at the time?' Perhaps we need to introduce a team of clinical ecologist lawyers to the bench in order to do tests to prove conclusively whether or not the prisoner in the dock is allergic in the manner he claims? See also **Aggression.**

VISION, DISTURBANCE OF

Symptoms affecting the eyes can have serious causes and medical advice must be sought early. Many different eye conditions exist which require early diagnosis and treatment. Foreign bodies in the eye can cause serious problems if not attended to rapidly, as can contact with chemicals. Some towns have their own eye hospitals.

Certain drugs used to treat mental depression and other conditions can cause side-effects which include blurred vision. Other visual upsets may be caused by drugs used to prevent fits. *Opren* is a drug which was used for arthritis; in some people, the drug was found to cause irreversible eye defects. A number of people so affected sued the company concerned and were compensated; the drug was removed from use.

A rare condition, night blindness, occurs when the eye fails to produce visual purple. This can be due to a lack of vitamin A.

Visual disorders can be of allergic origin. They can accompany a headache. A typical example of distortion of vision, as a symptom of allergy, is in migraine in which there may be split vision, half-vision, flashing lights, zig-zag lines or other visual disturbances. Conjunctivitis is a condition which may be caused by allergy or infection. It causes redness, watering of the eyes and very often blurring of the vision as a result.

All these allergy-related disturbances of vision are associated with eating certain foods, or food additives, or coming into contact with

V

chemical substances such as perfumes, cigarette smoke and so on. Colourings tartrazine (E102) and canthaxanthin (E161g) have been implicated with eye disorders. Inhalant allergens are also another possible cause of visual disturbance.

When I was trying to discover all the things to which I was allergic, I used to use the patterned tiles on my kitchen floor as a sort of barometer! The extent to which the pattern jumped about at any given time denoted how allergic I was. It could be a fascinating experience! I mentioned this to my optician and he explained that this is called 'retina rivalry' and if I closed one eye the pattern would stay still. I went home and found he was right, and was most impressed!

Supplements which will help eye problems, whatever the cause, are vitamins A and B complex, vitamin C and vitamin E.

V

WEIGHT LOSS

People who choose to lose weight – ie, those who go onto slimming diets – are recommended to lose no more than one to two pounds a week. Fats and sugars should be replaced, in the main, by cereals, bread, pulses, fruit and vegetables. Carbohydrates (bread and potatoes) are not in themselves fattening – it is what we add to them which causes the problems!

Anyone who wishes to slim would, undoubtedly, benefit from being more active. Regular, vigorous exercise of the type you enjoy is the answer. Start slowly and gradually work up to this, according to your age. If you have any heart or other problems, consult your doctor first.

Some people choose to lose weight but go too far, as in anorexia nervosa. They need professional help.

Fit people who do *not* choose to lose weight, but do so anyway, do not need to consult a doctor unless they are worried or their weight loss is excessive. Most of us change weight over the years for no apparent reason. The most annoying aspect of this, I think, is finding that your clothes do not fit as they should!

Those people who lose weight involuntarily, and are not well either, should obviously consult a doctor as weight loss can be symptomatic of many conditions, some serious. Sometimes an adverse reaction to food is involved, as in Crohn's disease and coeliac disease. Both cause weight loss due to lack of nutrients resulting from improper absorption of food from the gut.

The effects of caffeine (which is a drug) can effect a change in the metabolism which, in turn, can cause weight loss and other symptoms. This can result from taking excessive amounts of caffeine in any of its forms – coffee, tea, chocolate or cola – or from having developed a caffeine sensitivity, in which case even the most minute amounts may affect the susceptible individual. Other food allergies can cause weight loss, too; those referred to are simply the ones most commonly documented. In severe cases, patients have been known to lose weight with frightening rapidity – such as the lady recorded by Dr Richard Mackarness, in his book *Chemical Victims*, who lost twenty-five pounds in one month. This situation is likely to be reversed once the offending food is detected and eliminated from the diet. There are likely to be other symptoms which would make detection possible.

See also **Anorexia Nervosa, Coeliac Disease** and **Crohn's Disease**.

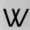

YAWNING

A common symptom of drowsiness. This can be related to physical, mental or emotional exhaustion or just plain boredom! It is not an unpleasant experience but can be most embarrassing if one cannot stop yawning when in the presence of others.

I cannot find any reference to yawning in relation to food or inhalant allergies but, obviously, any allergic reaction that causes a feeling of tiredness may cause someone to yawn. From my own experience it is my first sign of a reaction to cow's milk, but any food or inhalant could be responsible.

See also **Drowsiness** and **Tension/Fatigue Syndrome**.

ZOMBIE-LIKE STATE

In allergic people whose target area is the brain, the particular foods and chemicals to which they are sensitive can simulate the effects of drugs. The individual then begins to feel anything from drowsy or 'not with it' to total stupefaction. In this extreme state they will have as much difficulty in communicating with others as other will with them. However, do not be misled into thinking that they are not aware of what is going on around them. They are extremely sensitive to what is being said and quite conscious of the effect they are having. It is, however, just as if a sheet of plate glass had come down between them and the rest of the world. The ingrained routine, habits and obligations are so strong that such people will continue to perform as expected but in a totally mechanical manner. It is a very lonely and isolating experience.

My younger daughter went through a time of this silent suffering as a child before I realised that she was affected by citric acid. So keen had I been to ban orange squash with all its additives that I was making my own home-made brand which called for oranges, sugar and citric acid – which she was drinking daily!

All foods can cause this problem, especially the most common ones such as milk, wheat and eggs and, of course, artificial additives. The possibility of chemical inhalants should not be excluded. The most likely causes are the side-effects of drugs, especially anti-histamines such as *Piriton*.

See also **Brain Allergies, Drowsiness**.

USEFUL ADDRESSES

VOLUNTARY ASSOCIATIONS TO HELP MULTIPLE ALLERGY SUFFERERS

(Please enclose a stamped addressed envelope when sending for information.)

Action Against Allergy [Mrs P. Schooling]
24/26 High Street
Hampton Hill
Middlesex
TW12 1PD

Airedale Support Group [Mrs J. Wilson-Storey]
Briar Lea
Brookhouse
Nr Laughton
Sheffield S31 7YA
Tel: Dinnington (0909) 567929 (Ring preferably evenings and weekends)

Allergy Support Group, Oxford [Mrs V. Hibbert]
Lord's Cottage
2A Queen Street
Eynsham
Oxon OX8 1HQ
Tel: Oxford (0865) 883708 (Ring preferably between 4 and 6pm)

Cambridge Food Intolerance Society [Mrs K. Faruqi]
3 Stearne's Yard
Haslingfield
Cambridge CB3 7JA
Tel: Cambridge (0223) 871309

Chemical Victims [Mrs S. Hedges]
12 Highlands Road
Off Old Kempshott Lane
Basingstoke
Hants RG22 5ES
Tel: Basingstoke (0256) 465093

Hyperactive Children's Support Group [Mrs S. Bunday]
71 Whyke Lane
Chichester
West Sussex PO19 2LD
Tel: Worthing (0903) 725182
(Ring between 10.0am and 3.30pm, Tuesdays to Fridays inclusive)

USEFUL ADDRESSES

Hythe Food and Chemical Victims' Allergy Club [Mr J. Spells]
44 Fairview Drive
Hythe
Southampton
Hampshire SO4 5GY
Tel: Hythe (0703) 848902

Irish Allergy Treatment and Research Association Ltd
PO Box 1067
Churchtown
Dublin 14
Republic of Ireland

Levenmouth Allergy Support Group [Mrs E. Wallace]
10 Rannoch Road
Methil
Fife
KY8 3JD
Tel: (0333) 24247

Lothian Allergy Support Group [Miss J. Sturgeon]
19 Warrender Park Crescent
Edinburgh 9
(Or telephone Mrs E. Girling on 031 556 6924)

National Society of Research in Allergy [Mrs E. Rose]
PO Box 45
Hinkley
Leicester LE10 1JY
Tel: Hinkley (0455) 635212

Allergy Self-Help Group [Mrs Maureen Fairfield]
2 Roderick Avenue
Kirby in Ashfield
Notts NG17 9DB
Tel: (0623) 754358

Society for Environmental Therapy [Mrs H. Davidson]
521 Foxhall Road
Ipswich
Suffolk IP3 8LW
Scientific Society open to professionals as well as the lay public.

Sussex Allergy Support Group [Mrs Eva March]
15 Shermanbury Road
Worthing
West Sussex BN14 7HR
Tel: Worthing (0903) 208722

ASSOCIATIONS RELATED TO THE NEEDS OF ALLERGY SUFFERERS

Allergy-Induced Autism Support and Self-Help Group
Mrs Brenda O'Reilly
3 Palmera Avenue
Calcot
Reading
Berks RG3 7DZ
Tel: 0734 419460

Autism has been found in many instances to be related to food and chemical allergies. Mrs Brenda O'Reilly started AIA in 1988 since when it has made excellent progress gathering new members from both home and abroad. Among other things, they are very concerned about the use of chemical insecticides, herbicides and fungicides. After attention to diet, some of the children they represent have been able to go into mainstream schooling from special schools.

The Amarant Trust
14 Lord North Street
London SW1P 3LD
Tel: 071 222 1220

The Amarant Trust gives information and advice to women regarding hormone replacement therapy (HRT). Because of the overlap between hormones and allergies, some allergic women who have reached the change of life (or even before in some cases) may benefit from hormone replacement therapy. This is by no means a foregone conclusion, and full knowledge and understanding is essential before embarking on this treatment.

British Society for Allergy and Environmental Medicine
c/o The Burghwood Clinic
34 Brighton Road
Banstead
Surrey SM17 1BS

The British Society for Allergy and Environmental Medicine is concerned with the identification of patients suffering from food-allergic disease and the use of a dietary approach as the best means of treatment wherever possible. This method is used in conjunction with the detection of inhalant allergens, either natural or chemical, where it applies. The Society is open only to medical practitioners and the number of members is steadily increasing.

British Society for Nutritional Medicine
PO Box 3AP
London W1A 3AP

This newly established society deals exclusively with human nutrition as it relates to medical practice. Full membership is limited to qualified medical practitioners; associate membership is open to bona fide professionals such as nurses, biochemists, bona fide researchers etc and medical students. The Society holds a number of regular meetings on the practical aspects of nutrition both for general practitioners and hospital specialists.

Council for Involuntary Tranquillizer Addiction (CITA)
Cavendish House
Brighton Road
Waterloo
Liverpool L22 5NG

This Council is the headquarters which can provide information on clinics and self-help groups around the country, and which will be able to give help, advice and support to people wishing to come off tranquillizers. Please send a stamped addressed envelope when sending for information.

Food Additives Campaign Team
c/o The Food Commission
88 Old Street
London EC1V 9AR
Tel: 071 253 9513

The Food Additives Campaign Team (FACT) works very hard to protect our food from all additives which are known to produce, or are suspected of producing, harmful effects on our health. It has published an Additives Information Pack which is obtainable from the Publications Department at the above address.

Food Irradiation Campaign
The Food Commission
88 Old Street
London EC1V 9AR
Tel: 071 253 9513

Since the Government has decided to lift the ban on food irradiation we could have irradiated foods in the shops before the end of 1990. We were one of a minority of European governments who were in favour of irradiation – believing that it is a safe means of preserving foods and reducing the risk of food poisoning. The Food Irradiation Campaign is very concerned about this and calls for the current ban to remain in place until irradiation can be proven to be safe, wholesome and good for our food.

'Foresight' – Association for the Promotion of Preconceptual Care
Mrs P. Barnes
The Old Vicarage
Church Lane
Witley
Surrey GU8 5PN

'Foresight' is a well established scientific organisation which was formed to see that all possible steps were taken to ensure that every baby enters the world free from congenital deformity and mental damage and in perfect health. They advise on nutritional status in both prospective parents, protection from pollution, and how to reduce the chances of a child being born prone to allergies. They also do everything they can to instigate research into these and other potential hazards to foetal development.

Holiday Information
Mrs B. Hardcastle
40 Liebenrood Road
Reading
Berks RG3 2EB

Mrs Hardcastle, who is a member of the Basingstoke Association, Chemical Victims, has been collecting for some years now names and addresses of people offering holiday accommodation catering for the needs of food and chemical allergy sufferers. She will be pleased to furnish you with full information on receipt of a stamped addressed envelope. She is always pleased to hear of new places starting up.

ME Action Campaign
Director, Martin Lev
PO Box 1126
London W3 0RY

ME Action Campaign was started by a group of individuals who felt that a dynamic approach was required to solve the problems of ME. They have embarked on a medical research programme with the emphasis on non-drug treatments. This is a membership organisation with a network of groups nationwide which provide a range of services and information. They welcome new members but hear from too many people to be able to answer individual enquiries.

The Medic Alert Foundation
17 Bridge Wharf
156 Caledonian Road
London N1 9RD
Tel: 071 833 3034

The Medic Alert Foundation provides a prevention service that helps to keep people alive. It is estimated that every fifth person in this country has a hidden medical condition which could endanger their life in an emergency – diabetes, epilepsy, allergies and heart trouble, for example. The Medic Alert emblem, worn as a bracelet or necklet, is engraved with the wearer's special condition and twenty-four hour emergency telephone number.

National Childbirth Trust
9 Queensborough Terrace
London W2 3TV
Tel: 071 229 9319

A national organisation, with many local branches, that gives antenatal counselling to mothers-to-be and their partners. They teach relaxation methods and exercises, and they offer considerable post-natal support with advice on breast-feeding and other topics relating to caring for the newborn child.

USEFUL ADDRESSES

The National Pure Water Association
Secretary, Mr N. Brugge
Bank Farm
Aston Pigott
Westbury
Shrewsbury SY5 9HH

The National Pure Water Association has fought for many years against the compulsory fluoridation of water. It contends that, whereas chlorine and other chemicals are used to treat the water and make it safe to drink, fluoride is added to treat the water *consumer* and is an unacceptable infringement of the fundamental human right to decide for ourselves what substances (intended to affect the development of our bodies) go into our bodies.

Parents for Safe Food
Britannia House
1–11 Glenthorne Road
Hammersmith
London W6 0LS
Tel: 081 748 9898

Parents for Safe Food was started in 1989 to draw attention to health, environmental and economic problems associated with the use of pesticides, additives and other contaminants in our food. They are very concerned about bovine spongiform encephalopathy (BSE), and the possibility of food irradiation, and have produced fact sheets on both subjects. They want to help to ensure that we, as parents and consumers, have the choice of buying wholesome, uncontaminated food for our families.

Schizophrenia Association of Great Britain (SAGB)
Mrs Gwynneth Hemmings
Tyr Twr
Llanfair Hall
Caernarvon
N. Wales
Tel: 0248 670379

This well established scientific organisation promotes research into the biochemical causes of schizophrenia. Considerable help and support are given to sufferers and relatives with advice regarding possible dietary allergens which may be strongly linked with schizophrenia. A number of important scientific publications have been published through the Schizophrenia Association of Great Britain.

Soil Association
86 Colston Street
Bristol BS1 5BB
Tel: 0272 290661

The Soil Association operates an approval scheme for organic growers. Their symbol can be used only on food if it has been produced to the association's high standards. They publish regional lists (£2.50 each) and a national list (£10) of their approved growers. The prices include postage, and the lists are updated every six months.

GOODS AND SERVICES FOR ALLERGY SUFFERERS

Allerayde and Allergy Care Limited
1 Meadow Road
New Balderton
Newark
Nottinghamshire NG24 3BP
Tel: 0636 72636

Allerayde, which started in 1990, is a mail-order company specialising in a comprehensive range of environmental control products specifically designed to prevent exposure to house-dust mite in the home. These include bed covers, an allergy control spray, a vacuum cleaner filter and a room air-cleaner.

Allergy Care Ltd will offer RAST tests on pollens, animal furs, moulds, dust mites, drugs, chemicals and foods. Results of the tests will be evaluated by a doctor. They will stock a range of products, including those sold by Allerayde, plus allergen-free foods and specialist books. The first of a national chain opened in Nottingham during the autumn of 1990.

The Allergy Shop
2 Mount Place
Lewes
East Sussex BN7 1YH
Tel: 0273 472127

The Allergy Shop, a new mail-order company run by allergy-relief specialists, has been set up with the purpose of finding safer ways of meeting the everyday needs of the allergy sufferer. For their products they use only tried and tested ingredients of the purest quality. Their comprehensive range of products includes household materials and cleaners made from special formulations free from all harsh additives. Their toiletries are perfume- and lanolin-free, and they come packed in *glass* containers and include lotions of Oil of Evening Primrose. They offer a wide range of vitamin, mineral and nutritional supplements free from additives and animal products.

Almay
225 Bath Road
Slough
Bucks SL1 4AU
Tel: 0753 23971

Almay specialises in producing cosmetics for sensitive skins. As well as being unperfumed their products are free from ingredients that are known to act as irritants and include only minimal amounts of preservatives and anti-oxidants. They also produce a lanolin-free range of products for those allergic to lanolin. Their products are stocked in most large chemists and department stores and they will supply names of local stockists. A complete list of ingredients for all products is available to dermatologists.

Beta Plus
177 Haydons Road
Wimbledon
London SW19 8TB
Tel: 081 543 1142

Beta Plus stock a wide range of air purifiers which suck in the air and filter it in order to remove smoke, dust, pollen, mould spores and other potential allergens using an electrostatic filter. Running costs are relatively low. Their equipment can be seen in their showrooms or, if preferred, can be supplied by post.

Cantassium Co. Ltd (Larkhall Laboratories)
225–229 Putney Bridge Road
London SW15 2PY
Tel: 081 874 1130

This firm produces a wide range of additive-free vitamins and minerals, and many other supplements. They will give advice on what supplements would be the most suitable, taking into account individual allergens. They will send direct to customers and/or inform you of your nearest stockist. They sell a range of gluten-free, lactose-free and even grain-free flours. These are produced under the names Jubilee and Trufree and are obtainable at most chemists.

Cotton On
29 North Clifton Street
Lytham
Lancs FY8 5HW
Tel: 0253 736611

Cotton On produces all-cotton goods which are invaluable to people for whom wool and/or artificial fibres present a problem. They have a wide range of children's clothing in pretty colours and practical styles, including beach wear, underwear, pyjamas, jumpers, dungarees, T-shirts, tights and socks, boys' classic school shirts and trousers. For adults they stock jumpers, cardigans, stockings and tights etc. They also do a range of 100% cotton cellular blankets in all sizes. A leaflet illustrating their products will be sent on request.

Ecover
Mouse Lane
Steyning
West Sussex BN4 3DG
Tel: 0903 815614

Ecover produces a range of cleaning materials with the emphasis on biodegradability. However, as they use no enzymes, synthetic perfumes or colourings, they are also useful to people with contact or inhalant sensitivities. Their lavatory and bathroom cleaners contain no chlorine bleach.

Ecover products have been available for a number of years from health food shops. They are now being stocked by some of the leading supermarket stores.

Foodwatch International
Butts Pond Industrial Estate
Sturminster Newton
Dorset DT10 1AZ
Tel: 0258 73356

This is a mail-order service providing a wide range of foodstuffs especially tailored to the needs of allergy sufferers and others requiring special diets. Their services include a wide variety of unadulterated foods, cleaning materials and other items sent by mail order or carrier to any address in the UK or abroad, water purification systems to suit individual needs, and a technical advisory service on food composition, nutritional values, labelling etc. Customers are kept up-dated by regular copies of 'Food Watch News'.

Green Farm
Burwash Common
East Sussex TN19 7LX
Tel: 0435 882482

Green Farm provides a mail-order service free of charge which is normally despatched within twenty-four hours of receipt. They stock a wide range of products concentrating on quality, safety, absence of animal testing and friendliness to the environment. Their goods include ionisers, water purifiers, vitamin and mineral supplements, herbal preparations, skin, hair and bodycare preparations and aromatherapy oils. They also sell lambswool-filled duvets and pillows in pure cotton cases suitable for those who are sensitive to both feathers and synthetic fibres.

Norfolk Lavender Ltd
Caley Mill
Heacham
Kings Lynn
Norfolk PE31 1BR
Tel: 0485 70384

Norfolk Lavender is the only lavender farm left in England. Their delightful products include fragrances, soaps, bath products and lotions, sachets, dried lavender flowers and pretty Victorian gifts. A royalty is given to registered nature conservation charities. Their products are sold in pharmacies and gift shops but they offer a mail-order service for those who have difficulty in obtaining them.

Many people who find that they are sensitive to the chemicals used in many commercially produced scented goods will enjoy the pleasure of using these natural products.

Safe Homes and Buildings
Mr T. C. Hardwick
14 Rostrevor Mansions
Rostrevor Road
London SW6 5AP
Tel: 0424 853677, or 071 731 5202

This new company specialises in low-pollution housing. Its main aim is to advise allergy sufferers how to live as free from chemical allergens as possible. Mr Hardwick describes himself as a consultant and builder for the environmentally sensitive. He can give advice and specifications for building, decorating, adaptations, heating and ventilation, and will give advice on water purifiers, water filters, air filters, paints, varnishes, preservatives, waxes etc. Steam-cleaning of carpets and upholstery is another service he offers.

South Coast Environmental Services
22 London Road
Purbrook, Portsmouth
Hants PO7 5LJ
Tel: 0800 525781

This company specialises in environmental control. They produce dehumidifiers, humidifiers, heaters, coolers, air cleaners, air conditioners, blowers, fans and extractors. You can hire them, buy them or have them repaired. They don't come cheap, however. You may be more interested in air purifiers, ionisers and water filtration systems, which will provide clean, pollutant-free indoor air and water, thereby making your life pleasanter and healthier both in the short and long term. They stock them all and will be pleased to discuss your personal requirements.

MEDICAL SERVICES

Airedale Allergy Centre
Elmsley Street
Steeton, Keighley
West Yorkshire BD20 6SB
Tel: 0535 56013

The Airedale Allergy Centre is a purpose-built environmentally controlled allergy unit where allergy sufferers can go as in-patients or out-patients and be treated for food or chemical sensitivity. It is expensive, but every attention is given to patients' individual needs. The major medical insurance companies cover patients for this treatment. There are no NHS beds in the unit but a charitable trust has been formed which can help a small number of patients in financial need.

Allergy International
23 Edge Lane
Chorlton
Manchester M21 1JH
Tel: 061 881 0448

also:
Hale Clinic
7 Park Crescent
London W1
Tel: 071 631 0156

Allergy International has clinics in both Manchester and London. Their particular interest is in brain allergies but they cover a wide diversity of conditions and diseases of allergic and environmental origin.

Intradermal provocative skin testing and neutralisation in an allergy-free environment are used extensively for all forms of sensitivity. These include tests for foods, dust, dander and chemicals such as household gas and petrol fumes etc. Elimination dieting may be used where appropriate. Allergy International is recognised by BUPA, PPP and other medical insurance companies.

Biolab Medical Unit
The Stone House
9 Weymouth Street
London W1N 3FF
Tel: 071 636 5959/5905

The Biolab Medical Unit offers comprehensive nutritional testing and treatment for diseases in which nutrition plays a part. The tests they offer include sweat tests (for trace mineral balance), serum trace elements and toxic elements, B vitamins in blood and urine, vitamins A, C, E, carotene, amino acids, hair mineral profile and essential fatty acids. A medical referral is necessary for this treatment.

Biolab claims that their patients are covered by BUPA/PPP and other private health insurance companies, but BUPA declined to pay for my treatment on the grounds that: 'On checking our records we must advise that the Biolab Medical Unit is not on our list of recognised establishments.' I wrote to Biolab querying this and received no reply.

Breakspear Hospital
High Street
Abbots Langley
Herts WD5 0PU
Tel: 0923 261333

The Breakspear Hospital offers provision for both in-patients and out-patients who have become sensitised to food, air or water contaminants. It is a purpose-built environmental medicine hospital constructed within a beautiful old building. Only environmentally safe products, furnishings and materials have been used in its construction. Accommodation charges include all meals. Neutralisation treatment, pharmacy, pathology and patient management are extra. Charges are reviewed annually. It is costly, but every attention is given to patients' individual needs. The major medical insurance companies cover patients for this treatment.

Burghwood Clinic
34 Brighton Road
Banstead
Surrey SM7 1BS
Tel: 0737 361177/352245

The Burghwood Clinic is one of the few outpatient units in Great Britain specifically designed for diagnosing allergic and environmental illness. Initial investigation determines whether the patient's problem is predominantly food sensitivity, chemical sensitivity, inhalant sensitivity (house dust, dust mite etc), a yeast (*Candida*)-type condition, or a combination of these problems. Intradermal provocative skin testing and neutralisation therapy in an allergy-free environment are used extensively at the Clinic for all forms of sensitivity. Elimination dieting may be used where appropriate. The Burghwood Clinic is recognised by BUPA, PPP and other medical insurance companies.

London Medical Centre Allergy Unit
London Medical Centre
144 Harley Street
London W1N 1AH
Tel: 071 935 0023

The London Medical Centre Allergy Unit offers specialised assessment and treatment to patients with allergic disease – in particular asthma, eczema, hay fever, rhinitis, conjunctivitis, urticaria, irritable bowel syndrome and migraine.

Suitable patients are offered special treatment by enzyme-potentiated desensitisation (EPD). This method of treatment was discovered by Dr L. M. McEwen at St Mary's Hospital, London, in 1966. The technique was originally developed for the treatment of hay fever but has been extended to cover illnesses due to a wide range of inhalants and foods. A medical letter of referral is required, and the cost of treatment is generally covered by private health insurance.

Midlands Asthma and Allergy Research Association (MAARA)
12 Vernon Street
Derby DE1 1FT
Tel: 0332 362461/362462

The Midlands Asthma and Allergy Research Association is a registered charity formed in 1968 with the object of expanding research into the causes and treatment of asthma and all allergic disorders. MAARA also sponsors an Asthma and Allergy Treatment Clinic which provides a service for patients with allergic disorders such as asthma, rhinitis, hay fever, polyps, eczema, food sensitivity and urticaria etc. The clinic is recognised by BUPA and PPP etc, and referrals are made via the patient's GP. MAARA also provides an information service.

Premenstrual Tension Advisory Service
PO Box 268
Hove
East Sussex BN3 1RW
Tel: 0273 771366

The Premenstrual Tension Advisory Service provides advice which can bring about a natural resolution of symptoms. Their medical adviser specializes in nutritional medicine, in particular the nutritional approach to the premenstrual syndrome. A questionnaire is sent covering symptoms, diet, medical history, and lifestyle. Recommendations are based on the information you provide. It is advisable to check on current charges.

RECOMMENDED READING

Barnes, Belinda and Colquhoun, Irene. *The Hyperactive Child* (Thorsons, 1986)

Brostoff, Dr Jonathan. *The Complete Guide to Food Allergy and Intolerance* (Bloomsbury, 1989)

Button, John. *How to be Green* (Century Hutchinson Ltd, 1989)

Carson, Dr Paul. *How to Cope with Your Child's Allergies* (Sheldon Press, 1987)

Davies, Gwynn H. *Overcoming Food Allergies* (Ashgrove Press, 1985)

Davies, Dr Stephen and Stewart, Dr Alan. *Nutritional Medicine* (Pan, 1987)

Eagle, Robert. *Eating and Allergy* (Thorsons, 1986)

Edwards, Linda. *Baking for Health* (Prism Press, 1986)

Grant, Dr Ellen C. G. *The Bitter Pill* (Corgi, 1986)

Hanssen, Maurice. *E for Additives* (Thorsons, 1984)

Levin, Alan Scot. *The Allergy Relief Programme* (Gateway Books, 1985)

Mackarness, Dr Richard. *Not all in the Mind* (Pan, 1976)

Mackarness, Dr Richard. *Chemical Victims* (Pan 1980)

Mansfield, Dr John. *The Migraine Revolution* (Thorsons, 1986)

Mansfield, Dr John. *Arthritis: the Allergy Connection* (Thorsons, 1990)

Metland, Daphne. *A Pocketful of Es* (Foulsham, 1986)

Millstone, Eric and Abraham, John. *Additives: a Guide for Everyone* (Penguin, 1988)

Mindell, Earl. *The Vitamin Bible* (Arlington, 1986)

Moore, Pauline. *Milk-free, Egg-free Recipes for Children* (Foulsham, 1986)

Mumby, Dr Keith. *The Food Allergy Plan* (Unwin, 1985)

Mumby, Dr Keith. *Allergies: What Everyone Should Know* (Unwin, 1986)

Nathan Hill, Amelia. *Against the Unsuspected Enemy* (New Horizon, 1980)

Parents for Safe Food in association with the London Food Commission and Geoffrey Cannon. *Safe Food Handbook* (Ebury Press, 1990)

Parish, Professor Peter. *Medicines: a Guide for Everybody* (Penguin Books, 1987)

Rippere, Vicky. *The Allergy Problem* (Thorsons, 1983)

Rothera, Ellen. *Perhaps it's an Allergy* (Foulsham, 1988)

Scott, Sue. *Wholefood for the Whole Family* (Paperfronts, 1986)

Trickett, Shirley A. *Coming off Tranquillisers* (Thorsons, 1986)

Webb, Tony and Lang, Tim. *Food Irradiation – the Facts* (Thorsons, 1987)

White, Dr T. *Living with Allergies* (A Children's Book) (Franklin Watts, 1990)

Workman, Hunter and Jones, Alun. *The Allergy Diet* (Martin Dunitz, 1984)

RESEARCH

Unless indicated otherwise, the following passages are paraphrased from articles published in the medical journals cited. For more details, refer to the source cited.

Mygind, Niels. *An Illustrated Text for Students and Specialists* (Blackwell Scientific Publications, 1986)

'Despite the increase in our knowledge about allergy and the increase in public concern, the medical profession has been slow to absorb the new information which is available. Indeed, it is partly the neglect of the subject by the medical profession that has led patients to turn increasingly to the few practitioners, sometimes on the fringe of medicine, who are willing to spend their time on various ills that patients now regard as allergic.

In some ways we have a vicious circle. Many teachers of medicine know very little about allergy. If we do not find ways of including it in our educational system, many newly qualified doctors will be no better off and will share the limitations (and the prejudices) of their not very well informed teachers.'

Of the book, Lessof says: '... we should therefore welcome this excellent volume which will help to close the educational gap'.

Quoted from the book review by M. H. Lessof in *The Lancet* on 19 July 1986, p. 136.

Food Intolerance
Joint UK Databank Established

On 15 September 1987, the first Food Intolerance Databank was launched. It is based at Leatherhead Food Research Association. This will provide a unique service not found anywhere else in the world. Dietitians and hospital physicians will have access to data which will help in the treatment of food intolerance. The resources and experience of the British Dietetic Association, the British Nutrition Foundation, the Royal College of Physicians, the food industry and leading food and agricultural research institutes have been combined.

The major UK food companies have given details of the composition of over 4,000 food products. At first the databank will concentrate on the ten substances that the British Dietetic Association have found to be most problematic. These will include wheat and wheat derivatives, milk and milk derivatives, egg and egg derivatives, soya and soya derivatives, cocoa, sulphur dioxide, glutamate, benzoate, azo colours, butylated hydroxyanisole and butylated hydroxytoluene (BHA and BHT).

Because of recent increase in interest in food intolerance and the tendency to self diagnosis and treatment on unsuitable diets, access to the databank will be limited at first to dieticians and hospital physicians. The service will be provided free of charge.

The Lancet, 19 September 1987, p.677

Food Allergy in Idiopathic Nephrotic Syndrome
(Chronic disease of the kidneys where no organic cause can be found)

Dr Lagrue and colleagues studied adult INS patients with steroid failure in a search for signs of hypersensitivity to food. Twenty-six steroid-dependent INS patients were chosen. They did not necessarily have a history of food intolerance. Some foods were avoided on the basis of skin-tests, RAST 1gE and the human basophil degranulation test (HBDT). In six cases patients had complete and maintained remission, even after discontinuation of steroids.

In another study, Dr Lagrue and colleagues gave thirteen similar patients an oligoantigenic (hypoallergenic) diet for ten days whilst steroid treatment was maintained. In nine patients there was significant improvement with complete disappearance of symptoms in five of these cases. Soon after a return to a normal diet eight patients relapsed but remission was maintained in the other patient with exclusion of beef from the diet.

From their work, Dr Lagrue and his colleagues believe that food hypersensitivity may be a frequent occurrence in adult INS patients, even when clinical signs of food intolerance are absent. From this they suggest that food hypersensitivity may be more widespread than thought. (G. Lagrue, J. Laurent, G. Rostoker, P. Lang. Nephrology Service, INSERM Unit 139, Hospital Henri Mondor, 94010 Creteil, France.)

The Lancet, 1 August 1987, p.277

Penicillin Allergy in Childhood

An allergy to penicillin in children is over-diagnosed since, when tested with the drug, few such patients react adversely. The original diagnosis may be made on symptoms which have been produced for some other reason, such as an infection, eg, measles, a colouring agent (eg, tartrazine), preservative in the medicine or a viral infection.

Penicillin allergy may be caused by the 'major' determinant (which makes up about 95 per cent of the drug) or by 'minor' determinants (which make up the rest). The latter often lead to the severest allergies. There are three types of reaction. Immediate reactions occur within an hour of intake of the drug and are usually caused by the minor determinant. Symptoms include anaphylactic shock, bronchospasm, urticaria and laryngeal oedema. Accelerated reactions occur between one and seventy-two hours after administration and are usually caused by the major determinant. Similar symptoms are produced. Late reactions occur after seventy-two hours after administration and are less well understood. Symptoms include urticaria, rash, haemolytic anaemia, neutropenia and thrombocytopenia. Occasionally these reactions can be due to the development of an earlier reaction. Anyone suspected of penicillin allergy should not be given the drug since a reaction carries the risk of fatal anaphylaxis. A patient does not have to have a history of penicillin use since prior exposure and sensitisation can occur through penicillin encounters in food and drink.

The Lancet, 25 February 1989, p.420

Food Intolerance, Atopy and Irritable Bowel Syndrome

The cause of irritable bowel syndrome (IBS) is somewhat controversial. The degree to which food intolerance plays a part is considered debatable. Some researchers have suggested that hypnotherapy is effective, thereby implying a psychogenic origin for IBS.

Dr Smith and colleagues studied twenty-eight patients with IBS who had not responded to the usual treatment. Eleven patients were put on to a strict elimination diet. The only foods permitted were fresh white fish, lamb, peas, cabbage, carrots, milk-free margarine, *Ryvita* and weak, black tea. After a week there was a major improvement in two patients.

The remaining seventeen patients were put on the diet for two weeks and there was a significant improvement in nine cases. Those most likely to improve were patients with dominant diarrhoea. To identify specific food intolerances in the nine patients who responded, foods were reintroduced at two-day intervals. After a year, seven of these responders were still well as long as they avoided the foods to which they had been found to be intolerant.

The twenty-eight IBS patients were given prick tests to standard inhalant antigens. A matched control group without allergic disease had the same tests. The development of a wheal greater than 3mm to at least three antigens was defined as atopy. A significant difference in the percentage of patients who were atopic in both groups was found. Sixty per cent of IBS patients were atopic whereas only 23 per cent of the controls were. This suggests that IBS patients are unusually prone to allergy and is incompatible with the belief that IBS is of psychosomatic origin.

It was concluded, therefore, that IBS is an organic condition in which food intolerance plays a major part. Although there are several possible mechanisms of food intolerance, true food allergy may occur in some cases. Dr Smith and colleagues advise that IBS patients should be treated with standard techniques but that those who fail to respond should be offered an elimination diet for two weeks. (M. A. Smith, G. R. Youngs and Ronald Finn, Medical Units, Chester Royal Infirmary, Chester CH1 2AZ, and Royal Liverpool Hospital, Liverpool L7 8XP.)

Hunter, J. O. and Jones, V. A. *Food and the Gut* (Baillière Tindall, 1985)

The editors of this book describe in their preface their work at Addenbrook's Hospital in Cambridge on the treatment by diet of irritable bowel syndrome and Crohn's disease, although there is now evidence that diet is important in the management of other conditions such as migraine and eczema as well.

The nineteen chapters have been written, we are told, by many senior physiologists, microbiologists, gastro-enterologists and immunologists.

With regard to irritable bowel syndrome and Crohn's disease, an immunological explanation for these conditions seems unlikely and the editors suggest the reason may be the effect of dietary manipulation on microbial flora. To support this, they provide data showing how the use of antibiotics can lead to irritable bowel syndrome in women after hysterectomy. The editors clearly emphasise the interdisciplinary approach which is necessary for a good understanding of food intolerance and food-related disease. (Compiled from the review by Ann Ferguson, Gastro Intestinal Unit, Western General Hospital, Edinburgh)

The Lancet, 31 May 1986, p.1249

Coeliac Disease and Allergic Manifestations

Dr Hosker and colleagues in the November 15 issue of *The Lancet*, and Dr Hautekeete and colleagues in the January 17 issue of *The Lancet*, both looked at asthma and chronic urticaria as possible allergic manifestations of coeliac disease.

Dr Willliams took a detailed history of atopic disease and assessed pulmonary function of seventy-six adults with coeliac disease. Eighty-one control patients matched for age, sex and smoking with non-inflammatory bowel diseases were used. The former group had a significantly higher prevalence of airway obstruction, positive skin-prick tests to inhalants and foods and asthma. Incidence of eczema and rhinitis were similar in both groups. In ten out of the fifteen coeliac disease patients with asthma, the role of gluten in coeliac asthma was studied by giving oral gluten every day for three weeks and measuring pulmonary function. Asthma was reproduced in two patients but the immunological mechanism was not identified.

That asthma and urticaria are clearly associated with coeliac disease is not surprising since they are common symptoms of food sensitivity and intolerance. Other such symptoms which have been associated with coeliac disease include eczema, rhinitis, arthralgia, angioedema and migraine. Coeliac disease involves a true allergy to gluten. It has been suggested that coeliac disease could involve the formation of immune complexes, first in the small bowel and increased penetration of antigens through the mucosa. Dr Williams suggests that it is possible that symptoms such as urticaria and asthma could be caused by the release of mediators including histamine into the blood from the damaged small bowel. (Compiled from a letter by Alan J. Williams, Cardiothoracic Unit, Broadgreen Hospital, Liverpool L14 3LB.)

The Lancet, 4 April 1987, p.808

Food and Health

The Government is thought to be reluctant to make clear the ideals of healthy eating since if there was a major swing to consumption of foods of vegetable origin, high fibre, low saturated fat, salt and sugar, there would be less demand for subsidised surplus butter and farmers would suffer loss of revenue. However, the health of the nation would improve. Thus the consumer must gain information about healthy eating from sources other than the Government. Television has recently been a good source but such programmes tend to be watched by those who already have basic understanding of the problem. Books are also a good source.

The Lancet, 23 November 1985, p.1198

Food Safety

The potential hazards of food additives are attracting growing consumer concern. However, at the end of a report the Food Safety Research Consultative Committee has proposed that research into this area be cut back in favour of higher priority areas. Their explanation for this is lack of sufficient evidence of danger caused by food additives and contaminants in UK food. A more likely reason is that four out of the eleven committee members (including the Chairman) represent industrial interests. That this recommendation comes at the end of a report expressing regret at a planned decrease in funds for research into food safety, is strange to say the least.

The Lancet, 23 November 1985, p.1198

Food Labelling: Fat Only

The Government proposed mandatory labelling of food to display total fat and saturated fat content. Revised proposals for voluntary full nutritional labelling were circulated. The Government is thought to be trying to please both the health promotion lobby and the food industry which are in opposing camps.. Mandatory fat labelling does not give the consumer sufficient information to improve his diet. The Government intends full nutritional labelling to remain voluntary and it has suggested a standard format. However this format has been criticised by the Health Education Council for not distinguishing between starch, of which we should consume more, and sugar, of which we should consume less, which are both termed carbohydrate.

The Lancet, 22 February 1986, p.456

She Should Not Have Chewed

Tartrazine was the first food additive to be found responsible for side effects (reported in 1977) and it was followed by other azodyes, sodium benzoate, metabisulphites and butylated hydroxytoluene (BHT E321).

A young female had widespread urticaria which was not due to adverse drug reactions. Her only recent change of diet was the regular addition of chewing gum containing butylated hydroxytoluene. When the gum was omitted from use the eruption subsided within a week. Tests confirmed that BHT was, indeed, the problem. It is widely used as an antioxidant in foods such as potato crisps, salted peanuts, packeted cake mixes and dehydrated mashed potato. Oral provocation tests show that it can cause chronic urticaria. When looking for the causes of allergic symptoms, therefore, chewing gum should not be excluded. (Compiled from a letter from D. A. Moneret-Vautrin, M. C. Bene and G. Faure. Medicine D (Immuno-allergology) and Immunology Laboratory, UFR Sciences Medicales, CHU de Brabois 54500 Vandoeuvre-les-Nancy, France.)

The Lancet, 15 March 1986, p.617

Abram Ber, MD, FRCP(C), 'Neutralization of Phenolic (Aromatic) Food Compounds in a Holistic General Practice'. Quoted in full from *Journal of Orthomolecular Psychiatry* vol.12 no.4, fourth quarter 1983, p.283

'In September 1982, I attended the first symposium held at Brigham Young University on "The Immunotoxicity of Foodborne Phenolics and Airborne Pollutants".

The symposium was based on the findings of Dr Robert Gardner, PhD, Professor of Animal Science, Brigham Young University. Those practising alternative medicine will recognise the medical breakthrough of Dr Gardner's discovery and understand its overwhelming implications in the reversal of allergies and chronic degenerative diseases.

In 1979 Dr Gardener, a very allergic person, hypothesized that his allergies were caused by a sensitivity to some aromatic compounds found naturally in all plant foods and pollens. He acquired some of these pure aromatic compounds, made dilutions, started sub-lingual tests and monitored changes in pulse rates upon applications. There were reactions to various extracts and neutralizing doses were found for each compound. He found that neutralizing doses of these compounds would neutralize allergic reactions to specific foods. Months later, he had succeeded in neutralizing his own food allergies and he was now able to eat most foods without reactions. He gained weight lost during the years of sickness and felt a remarkable improvement in his health.

These aromatic food compounds naturally occur in all foods and are of small molecular weight. These compounds are not considered antigens but are likely haptens which probably become antigens after they gain entrance into the bodies of susceptible persons (McGovern et al, 1981).

Phenolics prolong the life and intensify cellular responses to catecholamines, causing cardiac stimulation and tachycardia. Peristalsis is increased in the intestine and distribution of blood is altered by these phenolics because of sensitizing smooth muscles to these catecholamines and other physiological stimulants. There is also increased entry of potassium ions into the cell under the influence of epinephrine (Fairbairn, 1959).

Once in the vascular system, phenolics may be conjugated in the liver and excreted back into the intestine via bile or eliminated in the the the urine.' (Written by Abram Ben M. D., FRCP(C), 3134N 7th Street, Phoenix, Arizona 85014.)

Change of Diet can Stop Migraine

A team of neurologists, dietitians and immunologists at the Hospital for Sick Children and Institute of Child Care, Great Ormond Street London, devised a treatment based on careful attention to diet. This was effective in reducing migraine attacks in children. They used eighty-eight subjects who suffered recurrent migraine attacks and eighty-two responded positively.

A strong link between migraine and certain foods, such as chocolate and cheese, has been shown by various groups, particularly those at the Princess Margaret Migraine Clinic and the City of London Migraine Clinic. Biochemical reactions stimulated by tyramine in these foods were thought to be responsible. Tyramine imitates adrenalin. However, regulation of tyramine levels did not support this theory. It is now suggested that migraine is food allergy. Extensive studies support this view.

A team of specialists, Dr J. Egger, Dr C. M. Carter, Dr J. Wilson, Dr M. W. Turner and Professor J. F. Soothill, put children onto a variety of diets for six months.

At first the children were given a simple diet. Foods were systematically added or removed if they led to symptoms. A group of children who were not prone to migraine followed the same procedure. Such a wide range of foods seemed to stimulate migraine – they identified a list of fifty-five – that it was concluded that this must be an allergic disease rather than a metabolic disorder.

The delay between consuming a food and the appearance of symptoms varied considerably. One child was allergic to twenty-four foods but, when these were excluded, suffered no symptoms. Often the children were particularly fond of the problematic foods, sometimes craving them. Most children reacted to cow's milk and all except one of them also reacted to cheese. (From an article by Pearce Wright, Science Editor.)

The Times, 2 November 1983, Home News

Roughness of Skin in Food Allergy

E. Cardi observed a high frequency of roughness of the skin in children with food allergy over many years of paediatric gastroenterology. He found dryness, roughness, goose bumps, keratosis pilaris and ichthyosis vulgaris. These changes occurred on the trunk, limbs and face. Dermatologists consider these signs to be 'stigmata associated with atopic dermatitis'.

Both children and adults with food allergy have been reported as having contact urticaria, generalised acute urticaria, chronic urticaria, swelling of the lips, rash, eczema, easy bruising and angioedema. But in our experience skin roughness and similar changes often occur in food allergy where atopic dermatitis or asthma may be absent. This has led to many correct diagnoses in the face of misleading clinical evidence.

We studied forty-six children aged between two months and fourteen years who had symptoms suggestive of food allergy. Forty patients responded to the elimination of cow's milk and its reintroduction after four to six weeks. Thirty-one patients (67 per cent) had rough skin and this occurred more often in children over three years. An equal number of age-matched patients without symptoms suggestive of food allergy were used as controls. Only four (9 per cent) had roughness of the skin. (Compiled from a letter E. Cardi, S. Lucarelli, T. Frediani, M. Barbato, A. Zingoni and P. De Gregorio, Department of Paediatrics, University of Rome, 'La Sapienza' 00161 Rome, Italy.)

The Lancet, 16 April 1988, p.886

Comprehensive Health

The first link between orthodox and complementary medicine in Britain was the health centre due to be opened in 1987 in the crypt of St Marylebone Church, London NW1. Here patients can consult an NHS general practitioner, an alternative practitioner (eg, an acupuncturist, osteopath, spiritual healer etc) or a religious counsellor. The centre operates as any other general practice for the local population but also takes referred patients from elsewhere. A preventive health care programme is available, involving medication, breathing, relaxation, diet and exercise. Research into holistic medicine will also take place. There will be no charge for NHS patients but some contribution is expected for other services.

The Lancet, 5 April 1986, p.814

Food Additives

The industrial and commercial use of food additives is controlled by the Ministry of Agriculture, Fisheries and Food, advised, in this case, by the Food Advisory Committee. Additives are considered firstly on need (eg colouring, flavouring, shelf-life extension) and secondly on safety. These safety aspects are considered by committees of the DHSS, largely the committee on toxicity but also those covering carcinogenicity and mutagenicity. The committees have their work covered by the Official Secrets Act. Dr Erik Millstone of Sussex University has written a book entitled *Taking the Lid off what we Really Eat* (Penguin Books, 1986). He raises serious doubts about the adequacy of safety testing of additives.

The Lancet, 5 April 1986, p.814

Water in Food

A report by the London Food Commission (now the Food Commission) shows that increasing amounts of water are being added to some types of food such as frozen fish, poultry and some cooked meat products. This is quite legal. Fish fingers, for example, now contain an average of around 55 per cent fish, though some samples were as low as 45 per cent compared to 60 per cent in 1970. Increased water content is largely responsible for the difference. The water is held in place by phosphate additives. The London Food Commission states that the 5 per cent extra water content of fish fingers represents a loss of three million pounds to the consumer and a corresponding gain by the retailers.

The Lancet, 18 July 1987, p.170

The Content of Processed Food

There has been a move to reduce fat intake by many people, especially saturated animal fats. Professor Geoffrey Rose (Department of Epidemiology, London School of Hygiene and Tropical Medicine), at a press conference on 3 December by the Coronary Prevention Group (CPG), pointed out that the fat content of food is not always clear to the consumer. He emphasised that in order to continue reducing the fat content of our food we need to be provided with the full nutritional breakdown of all processed foods.

The CPG has made a report on food labelling. In February, 1986, the Ministry of Agriculture, Fisheries and Food (MAFF) made the labelling of fat content (total and saturated) of food mandatory. However the Government states that compulsory, general nutritional labelling is against the EEC law and therefore impossible. Voluntary guidelines on methods of nutritional labelling were issued by MAFF in July 1986. The CPG is against these guidelines, even if they were made mandatory, since it is virtually impossible to make nutritional comparisons of different products. Also, the labelling of fibre, sugar and salt is not guaranteed. A barrister, Ms Anyadike-Danes, has argued against the Government's interpretation of the EEC's Food Labelling Directive. The CPG has asked the Government to clarify its position on nutritional labelling. Also, in view of Britain's very high number of deaths from coronary heart disease, it has called for proper and compulsory labelling of saturated fats, sugars, salt and fibre in processed foods.

The Lancet, 12 December 1987, p.1412

Hypothesis. Xenogeneic Antibodies and Atopic Disease

Xenogeneic antibodies can be absorbed through the human gut. They can withstand food processing and their activity may even be enhanced by such procedures. They function as antibodies and antigens in the human immune system. Dr Collins suggests that the human immune system is primed by low level exposure to xenogeneic antibodies, specific for human allergens common to farms, such as moulds, mites and pollens, resulting in an inappropriate response when these allergens are later encountered. In the western diet, the largest source of xenogeneic antibodies is dairy products. Dr Collins' hypothesis may partly explain the link between cow's milk and allergies to substances other than milk proteins. (Compiled from the Summary of a Hypothesis by Andrew M. Collins, Department of Genetics and Human Variation, La Trobe University, Bundoora, Victoria, Australia 3083.)

The Lancet, 2 April 1988, p.734

Contact Allergy to Self-Adhesive Dressings

A history of drug allergy is usually taken from patients admitted to hospital. However, this is not the case for adhesive dressings. Patients should be asked whether they are allergic to *Elastoplast*, as adhesive dressing is almost always used after surgical procedures. One patient did tell his surgeon of his allergy but he was told that *Transpore* (3M) would not cause a problem. The allergen in *Elastoplast* is colophony, which is also present in *Transpore*. Good alternatives which omit colophony are *Micropore* (3M) and *Dermalite* (Johnson and Johnson). (Compiled from a letter from Colin Hindson and Susan Sinclair, Department of Dermatology, Royal Infirmary, Sunderland SR2 7JE.)

The Lancet, 28 May 1988, p.1224

Halothane Allergy as Cause of Acne

Dr Guldager suggests that the appearance of acne in operating theatre staff should be considered as a possible halothane allergy. Although this link has previously only been described in one case, he believes halothane allergy could be a hidden problem for operating theatre staff. He describes another case of a twenty-seven-year-old woman who had acne on her face two weeks after starting work as a nurse anaesthetist. No relief was given by use of a steroid cream or tetracycline. Four months later she administered a halothane anaesthetic and had eruptions over her whole body. She was diagnosed as having an allergic skin reaction but there was no liver involvement. The nurse was transferred to work on an intensive care unit. Whenever she comes into contact with a patient who has just had an anaesthetic involving halothane, she develops widespread acne within a few hours. (Compiled from a letter from Henrik Guldager, Department of Anaesthesiology, Hvidovre Hospital, 2650 Hvidovre, Denmark.)

The Lancet, 23 May 1987, p.1211

Chronic Urticaria Associated with Coeliac Disease

Hosker and colleagues (Hosker, H. S. R., Kelly, C. A., Bird, G., Clague, H. and Walkers E. H.: Adult coeliac disease presenting with symptoms of worsening asthma, *Lancet* 1986, ii, 1157–8) reported two patients with asthma and adult coeliac disease who showed marked improvement in respiratory symptoms on a gluten-free diet.

Dr Hautekeete and colleagues report a patient with chronic urticaria and adult coeliac disease whose urticaria disappeared on a gluten-free diet. He is a forty-seven-year-old man who had generalised urticaria which did not respond to drug treatment. He gained weight on a gluten-free diet, and the urticaria started improving after two months and disappeared after three months. There was no recurrence following a year on a gluten-free diet. Atopic disorders (asthma, eczema and hay fever) are also clearly associated with coeliac disease. It has been suggested that atopy in coeliac disease is the result of allergens passing through the damaged mucosa. They conclude that coeliac disease should be considered when investigating chronic urticaria. (Compiled from a letter from Marc L. Hautekeete, Luc S. De Clerck and Wim J. Stevens, Department of Clinical Immunology, Antwerp University Hospital, Antwerp, B-2520, Belgium.)

The Lancet, 17 January 1987, p.157

Food Allergy and Dyspepsia

Drs Canonica and Ciprandi refer to Dr Colin Jones' report (12 March, p.576) of the helpful suggestions of a group of ten gastroenterologists on the management of dyspepsia. Food allergy, they say, has been considered as a possible, though almost irrelevant, causative factor in some dyspeptic symptoms. For their part they wish to highlight some points about the mechanisms connecting dyspepsia and food allergy and about the incidence of this symptom in individuals with adverse reactions to foods.

They have observed about twenty per cent of dyspeptic symptoms in more than 200 patients with the urticaria angioedema syndrome due to food intake. Improvement obtained from drugs with a cytoprotective activity on the gastro-intestinal mucosa has been noted. The three cytoprotective agents they used were pirenzepine, rosaprosol and sucralfate together with classical antihistamines. The results were excellent when compared with other drugs. This points to the importance of looking for a possible allergic mechanism (primary or not) in patients with dyspepsia and vice versa. (Compiled from a letter from G. Walter Canonica and Giorgio Ciprandi, Department of Internal Medicine, University of Genoa, 16132, Genoa, Italy.)

The Lancet, 28 May 1988, p.1233

Index

Bold numbers indicate the main entry.